Stammer
and Prejudice

British Library Cataloguing in Publication Data

A catalogue record for this book is available from the British Library

Cover design: Jim Wilkie

Cover image : Kirsten Hinte used under license from Shutterstock.com

Project management, typesetting and design: J&R Publishing Services Ltd, Guildford, Surrey, UK; www.jr-publishingservices.co.uk

Printed and bound by CPI Group (UK) Ltd, Croydon, CR0 4YY

Stammering Pride and Prejudice

Difference not Defect

Patrick Campbell, Christopher Constantino
and
Sam Simpson (Eds)

J&R Press Ltd

Contents

Acknowledgements

Together Patrick, Chris and Sam would like to thank all those connected with the book, however tangentially. Our most heavy-hearted thank you goes to Mike Oliver. A titan of disability studies, Mike was encouraging and supportive after we reached out to him, rather out of the blue, to write a foreword for us. Mike sadly died in March 2019. The grief felt in the disabled community after his loss reflects not only the lasting power of his work, but also the inherent goodness of the man behind it.

We would also like to pay tribute to David Mitchell, one of the greatest authors of our age, whose generous offer of time to write a foreword validated our belief in this book's worth. His speech 'Thirteen ways of looking at a stammer' remains an ongoing source of inspiration.

We thank Rachael and Jim Wilkie, our publishers, for taking a punt on a different kind of stammering book. The social model of disability has little track record in stammering. Most prominent research and publications in the field are still based on a medical model perspective. Rachael and Jim, as well as providing technical and professional skills, bravely believed in us and valued the importance of the radical ideas we wanted to express.

We would also like to thank our tireless and generous contributors, authors and artists. They have given their time, energy and a part of themselves to this book freely. Their words, drawings, pictures and poetry have challenged and inspired us as editors.

We owe debt of gratitude to Skype, Google Docs, and Dropbox for enabling a seamless transatlantic collaboration. We also owe a debt to the wider stammering community who have inspired the ideas within this book and to you, dear reader, for taking the time to engage with them. We can only hope you have as much joy reading this book as we did editing.

Patrick would like to thank: his friends and family, for being there for him; Chris and Sam, for their friendship, company and wisdom; the contributors, for their hard work, generosity and insight; and the stammering community, for their support and solidarity.

Chris is thankful to God for creating him with a stutter. He is grateful for the endless patience, intelligence, and kindness of his wife, Megan. He is also grateful for Megan's refried beans, butternut squash soup, and peanut butter

& fig cookies, which fuelled the editing of this book. He appreciates the love and support of his parents, brothers, and sisters. He appreciates his bicycle for the time it has given him to reflect, ponder, and meditate on this book's ideas. He is grateful for his co-editors, for Sam's nuance and sensitivity and Patrick's brevity and sensibility but, most of all, for their levity and friendship.

Sam would like to acknowledge: her co-editors, Patrick and Chris, of whom she has become very fond throughout the lengthy and at times intense editorial process. She thanks them both for the technical wizardry, generosity and good humour they have brought to the project. Finding kindred spirits committed to questioning and challenging established norms and therapeutic practices in relation to stammering has been healing, expanding and energising; Thierry, for his steady presence, flexibility and encouragement; Elise, Amy and Anouk for keeping her grounded and connected to what she values most in life; to all her friends and colleagues for their unique contributions over the years to her becoming the person and the therapist she has become; and finally to the many people who stammer who have touched her life and taught her the importance of looking beyond the assumed.

About the Contributors

Emma Alpern grew up in Pennsylvania and currently lives in Brooklyn, New York, where she works in the publishing industry. She is a fan of stuttering communities, the National Stuttering Association conference and support groups, and stuttering activism. She has blogged about her speech at stuttermore. tumblr.com.

Katy Bailey is now a very contented stammerer. Her circuitous career has involved work in mental health, participatory research in disability studies, being a mum and back to mental health. Her consistent interest is in what we can do and be when we are together in groups; she is passionate about Peer Support, how people share experience, theorize and produce knowledge together, and she is a group worker with Mind in Leeds. Katy (and those around her) benefits from her commitment to mindfulness and meditation. She has recently learnt to row and loves looking out for kingfishers whilst getting a workout.

Nisar Bostan never got back to us with a biography. For those of us who have the pleasure of knowing Nisar, this seems in a way in keeping with who he is: an undefinable, quirky and brilliant human.

Michael Boyle is an Associate Professor in the Department of Communication Sciences and Disorders at Montclair State University. He teaches graduate courses in fluency disorders and conducts research on psychosocial aspects of stuttering, such as stigma and empowerment.

Patrick Campbell is a stammerer and junior doctor living in Cambridge, England. He has an interest in how public- and self-stigma intertwine to produce disability for people who stammer and how this debilitating process can be altered through seeing positive value in stammering. Recently, Patrick has enjoyed taking part in local 5k runs.

Carolyn Cheasman has worked with adults who stammer at City Lit, London since 1979. She has experienced interiorized stammering herself and so brings both personal and professional interests to the field. Having completed post-qualification training in personal construct psychology and person-centred counselling, she went on to train as a mindfulness teacher and now teaches mindfulness to people who stammer, speech and language therapists and the general public. In 2012, Carolyn was honoured to receive the International

Fluency Association Clinician of Distinction award. She became interested in the influence of the social model of disability in the late 1990s and has been involved in the development of self-advocacy groups at City Lit.

Christopher Constantino lives in Tallahassee, Florida with his wife Megan. He is a speech-language pathologist and assistant professor at Florida State University. He teaches classes on counselling and stuttering and researches how the lived experience of stuttering interacts with culture and society. Chris enjoys making and eating ice cream and riding his bike.

Rachel Everard is a specialist speech and language therapist whose decision to train as a therapist stemmed from the fact that she stammers herself and from her life-changing experience of receiving therapy at City Lit. After qualifying in 1996, she worked in a variety of settings including community clinics and mainstream primary schools before joining the City Lit team in 2001. In 2019, she took up a new post as Service Director at the British Stammering Association. Due to her own personal experience of stammering, she strongly believes in empowering people who stammer and in the importance of developing stammering communities as well as educating the general public about stammering.

Nina G is a comedian, professional speaker, storyteller, writer and educator. She brings her humour to help people confront and understand Disability culture, access, and empowerment. Nina shares her wit and wisdom with corporations, colleges, community/Disability awareness events and media interviews. Nina is author of *Stutterer Interrupted* and *Once Upon an Accommodation*.

Doreen (Dori) Lenz Holte is mom to a 23-year-old son who stutters and author of *Voice Unearthed: Hope, Help, and a Wake-up Call for the Parents of Children Who Stutter* (www.voiceunearthed.com). Dori enjoys connecting with parents across the world on the Voice Unearthed Facebook group and with students, professional organizations, and speech therapy groups. She also enjoys doing grant consulting work for nonprofits, teaching grant writing workshops, and playing card and board games with her family. She recently took up tap dancing.

Kristel Kubart is a speech language pathologist who has cerebral palsy and who stutters. Growing up with two disabilities has had a major impact on her experiences in the world and her place in it. She has a passion for working with children, teens, and adults who stutter. Kristel currently works for the

American Institute for Stuttering (AIS) and in the New York City public schools. She has led numerous workshops and trainings for other speech therapists and people who stutter and their families at organizations like the National Stuttering Association (NSA) and FRIENDS (The National Association for Young People Who Stutter). In her spare time, she likes to do Pilates, make art, and travel. In the future, Kristel plans to get more involved in the cerebral palsy community.

Grant Meredith is an academic and futurist within the School of Science, Engineering & Information Technology at Federation University Australia. He leads the applied Technologies for Empowering People for Participation in Society (TEPPS) research program, where he enjoys making assertive technologies to empower people who stutter.

David Mitchell is the award-winning and bestselling author of *The Thousand Autumns of Jacob de Zoet*, *Black Swan Green*, *Cloud Atlas*, *Number9Dream*, *Ghostwritten* and *The Bone Clocks*. Twice shortlisted for the Man Booker Prize, Mitchell was named one of the 100 most influential people in the world by *TIME* magazine in 2007. With KA Yoshida, Mitchell co-translated from the Japanese the international bestselling memoir, *The Reason I Jump*. He lives in Ireland with his wife and two children.

Mike Oliver obtained his BA (Hons) Sociology and Social Anthropology at University of Kent in 1975 and his PhD in 1979. He then worked as a lecturer at the University until 1982 before moving on to be a senior lecturer in special educational needs at Avery Hill College. In 1991, he became the first Professor of Disability Studies in the United Kingdom at the University of Greenwich and worked there until his retirement in 2003. Mike co-founded the international journal of *Disability and Society* and was an executive editor until his retirement. He was an internationally recognized academic and political commentator, having participated in several major policy reviews in education, health and social services and published numerous books and articles on disability and other social policy issues over the last 30 years. Mike also made many appearances on national and regional television and radio. He was an active member of the Disability movement and worked with many organizations of disabled people. He spent his free time supporting Arsenal, investing in the betting markets and listening to the music of Bob Dylan and Leonard Cohen. Mike Oliver sadly died on 2 March 2019. He left behind a wife, two grown-up children and two grandchildren.

Ann Packman is Professor of Speech Pathology at the Australian Stuttering Research Centre, University of Technology Sydney, Australia, and has over 40 years' experience working with people who stutter. She has over 200 publications on stuttering, comprising journal papers and books. Ann is currently on the Advisory Board of the Australian Speak Easy Association and, together with members, she conducts forums each year for student teachers on how they can support children who stutter in the classroom.

Zahari Richter is a PhD student of English, focusing on Contemporary American Literature and Media, at George Washington University. In their free time, Zahari enjoys Pokemon Go and hiking.

Wendy Ronaldson is studying for a BA Fine Art Degree at University Centre Grimsby and has lived with a stammer from the age of 5 years. Wendy has contributed to British Stammering Association conferences by offering talks and creative workshops related to speech and language issues. Wendy enjoys being creative through her artwork using various techniques and methods to create different forms.

Erin Schick is a social worker living in New York. Their work focuses on queer liberation and disability justice. Erin is passionate about outdoor recreation, women's soccer, and healthcare policy.

Walter Scott is a civil servant, Government communications specialist, and co-founder of the Defence Stammering Network. He has written and spoken extensively on stammering and societal attitudes, publishing some of this material in an e-book, *A Few Quick Words: Outspoken Thoughts on Stammering*. He has worked with Forces TV on two documentaries – *My War with Words* (2014) and *Stammering: The Unspeakable Truth* (2018) – appeared on BBC 5 Live, and delivered a TEDx talk entitled 'Life with a stammer'. His interests include parenting, allotmenteering, percussion, and unearthing long-forgotten Victorian painters.

Sam Simpson is a speech and language therapist and person-centred counsellor (www.redefiningstammering.co.uk). Sam co-edited *Stammering Therapy from the Inside: New Perspectives on Working with Young People and Adults* with Carolyn Cheasman and Rachel Everard. She works in independent practice and contributes to the development and delivery of the professional training programmes offered by the City Lit speech therapy team, intandem and Metanoia Institute. In her free time, Sam enjoys walking her dog, singing in a choir and mindfulness meditation.

Joshua St. Pierre holds a PhD in philosophy from the University of Alberta. He specializes in critical disability theory at the intersection of contemporary political, feminist, and communication theory. The overarching theme of his research is a critique of fluency. He has numerous academic publications on speech disabilities, the history of Speech-Language Pathology, eugenics, and feminist theory. Joshua is also a co-founder of the *Did I Stutter* project, an activist community created by and for stutterers to embrace dysfluent voices and raise awareness of speech discrimination.

Josh Walker studied medicine at the University of Manchester and is now a junior doctor in Northern Ireland. He has a stammer and has been involved with City Lit and British Stammering Association (BSA) groups for a number of years. His interest in social theory began when studying a Global Health BSc, culminating in a dissertation that explored the cultural limitations of modern psychiatry. He has gone on to develop an interest in therapy, exploring narrative-based and person-centred approaches in particular.

Iain Wilkie is an experienced mentor and executive coach who stammers (www. iainwilkie.com). Using experience gained from his 21 years as a partner in the professional services firm Ernst & Young (EY), he is committed to supporting all people who stutter to achieve their full potential in their work. Iain is the founder of the EY Stammering Network, the UK's Employers Stammering Network and 50 Million Voices. He enjoys outdoor activities, such as walking, cycling and watching rugby, as well as singing in a local choir.

Sarah Wilkinson is a musician, educator and writer from West Yorkshire. She is a person who stammers. In 2018, she published her first children's book *All in a Day* and is working towards more publications for children and adults in the near future.

Elizabeth Wislar is a person who stutters and a teacher of students with disabilities. She lives in Athens (Georgia, USA) with her husband, daughter and a multitude of pets. She loves to run, cook, draw, read and write. She is the leader for the Athens National Stuttering Association chapter and writes a blog about being a teacher who stutters (https://thestutteringteacher.wordpress. com/). She feels strongly that people with disabilities deserve equality and believes her stutter to be an asset and a strength.

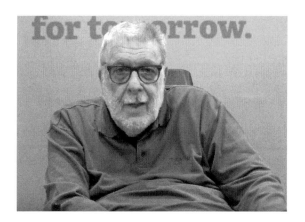

Foreword

Mike Oliver
Emeritus Professor of Disability Studies

When, nearly 40 years ago, I named a radical set of ideas about disabling barriers and environments *the social model of disability*, I really had no idea people would still be using it and writing about it today. It was never intended to be anything other than a device to get my students thinking about how they might apply these ideas when working with disabled people.

However, the social model quickly became the mechanism for raising political consciousness amongst disabled people and served as a gold standard for judging economic and social policies affecting disabled people. Thus, it was adopted by policymakers and politicians not just in the United Kingdom but in many other countries as well. Many disability organizations also endorsed it.

Success usually brings criticism with it as well and one of the major ones was that it was easy to see how the model applied to wheelchair users but that it was less clear how it might be applied to other impairments, especially non-visible, sensory and cognitive ones. My response was to point out that it was never intended to be applied to all disabled people and all of their personal circumstances and relationships with the worlds in which they lived.

I always saw the social model as a device to help disabled people to make sense of what was happening to them individually or collectively and a tool to help them overcome the barriers they were facing regardless of what kind of impairment they had. Some seven years after I had introduced the social model, as a rejoinder to some of its critics, I used the specific example of stammering to point out that it could be utilized by a range of different impairment groups to improve the lives they were living.

Thirty years later, I was delighted to receive an invitation to write a foreword to this book because it not only applies the social model of disability to understanding the lives of people who stammer but also serves as a political impetus to improving these lives. I earnestly hope that people who stammer find it as empowering as other impairment groups have in our quest to take our rightful places in the worlds in which we live and remove many of the barriers we all face.

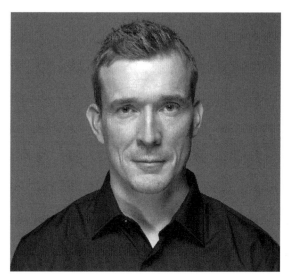

Photo by Paul Stuart

Foreword

David Mitchell
Award-winning author and stammerer

My 'method' for writing forewords is to read the book or e-manuscript with a sheet of A4 and pen in my hand and jot down a Top 10 of eye-catching quotes, or mind-catching ideas, which I then structure my foreword around. By the time I reached the middle of *Stammering Pride and Prejudice*, however, my method had failed: I was on my fifth sheet of A4, and was transcribing whole chunks of this excellent book line by line. To read *Stammering Pride and Prejudice* is to be party to a conversation about speech disfluency and disability – a conversation as informed, intelligent and diverse as any I've known. The range of contributors is startling. In the following pages, you'll meet a doctor who stammers; the mother of a child who stammers; a young woman with cerebral palsy who stammers; poets and artists who stammer; a teacher who stammers; speech pathologists who stammer; activists, advocates and 'resistors' who argue, persuasively, that the very notion that stammering is a 'pathology' is a part of the problem. You'll encounter angles on speech disfluency that would never occur to a non-insider, such as the battles with Siri and voice-operated phone menus; and the phenomenon of self-stigma. This brief list, literally, isn't the half of it.

Editors Patrick Campbell, Christopher Constantino and Sam Simpson deserve congratulations not only for assembling such a worthwhile group of contributors, but for curating a conversation with respect for differing viewpoints – a courtesy so sorely lacking in public and online discourse elsewhere. *Stammering Pride and Prejudice* has no agenda beyond a deeper, smarter and kinder understanding of stammering in particular and disability in general. This approach is particularly appropriate for stammering, which is so chock-full of contradictions and paradoxes. Is stammering a curse? Is it a gift? Should we try to eliminate it? Or should we eliminate the notion that it needs eliminating? What causes it? Up which tree should we be barking? Is it genetically triggered? Is it environmentally aggravated? Is it the stammer that's the problem, or the society that stigmatises and isolates stammerers? By giving space to opposing ideas, by acknowledging all may have merit, the editors have created an ecosystem of ideas far more fertile than the monoculture of a single argument that conquers all others.

Reading *Stammering Pride and Prejudice* has made a much better-informed stammerer of me. I found myself questioning prejudices that I'd never noticed. I groaned, retrospectively, at blunders of thought and deed that contributors brought to my attention. I laughed, surprisingly often. I was moved by people's bravery, knowing – first-hand – that this bravery often feels like abject failure. I was moved by people's honesty, and admiring at how they shared painful experiences for the benefit of strangers. I clucked my tongue in recognition at certain situations, embarrassments and gambits. I felt less alone. A few times, I welled up. My curiosity was energised and my understanding was enriched, as if I had attended a campus open day at a Faculty of Stammering Studies in a University of Being a Better Human.

I'd like to wind up this brief foreword with just one of the quotes from my scrawled A4 sheets, by the contributor Zahari Richter:

> 'I dream of a day when all stutterers are taught that there is nothing wrong with them and that it does not matter how long it takes you to say a word or how many misunderstandings you have in daily conversations and to instead realize that what matters is the effort you put in and the spirit in your everyday expressions.'

This quote, like the book in which it is housed, is an invitation to rethink and redraw our inherited map of speech disfluency. To my mind, there *is* room for speech therapy on this map; but equally, speech therapy is not the map's entirety. The essays, accounts, research, prose, testimonies, art and poetry in this multidisciplinary anthology will nourish and inform readers who stammer, and readers who don't, for many years to come. Whether a stammer is a pathology, a quirk to be celebrated, a curse or a blessing, or all these things, *Stammering Pride and Prejudice* is a gift.

David Mitchell
July 2019

Our fortnightly Skype
meeting on Mondays
at 20.30 GMT!

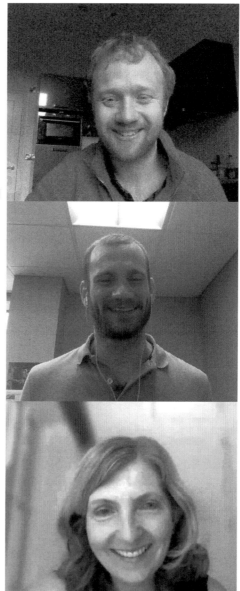

Patrick Campbell

Christopher Constantino

Sam Simpson

Introduction

Patrick Campbell, Christopher Constantino and Sam Simpson

Back in 1974, the Canadian rock group Bachman-Turner Overdrive were compiling their third album. Charlie Fach, a producer for Mercury Records, reviewed their proposed collection of eight songs. Fach was not convinced. He thought it lacked a potential hit song and, in particular, he 'couldn't hear the magic'. The band had another song recorded. An instrumental piece with lyrics written on the fly, it was sung in stammered vocals to poke fun at the band's former manager who stammered. Out of other ideas, they played it to Fach. Fach liked it. "That's the track! It's got a brightness to it. It kind of floats a foot higher than the other songs when you listen to it."

Bachman-Turner Overdrive re-recorded the song to include it in the album, but sung with fluent vocals. It did not work. With the stammering removed, the magic was lost. They decided to keep the stammering and the rest is history. What was once a joke became a chart-topper in six different countries and can still be heard on the airwaves today.

Stammering is often seen as a joke and it is taken for granted in our society that fluency is better than stammering. But, as the story of 'You Ain't Seen Nothing Yet' reminds us, this is not necessarily true. Stammering can benefit both people who stammer and society if we let it.

This book is a collection of voices that live and breathe this idea. It has been a long time coming.

Beginnings

Stammering Pride and Prejudice was born out of our shared frustration with the thin and negative understandings of stammering available to people who stammer. We live in a society which stigmatizes stammering. Sometimes this stigma becomes active discrimination, such as when a stammerer is mocked or denied a job. However, often it is more insidious. At its most potent, it operates as taken-for-granted assumptions about the inferiority of stammering; that being fluent is somehow *better* than stammering. If you told your neighbour you were going to stammering therapy to become fluent, they would not think anything of it. But if you told them you were going to therapy to stammer more, likely they would be rather confused. Stigma makes the sentence "I wish I was more fluent" banal and the sentence "I wish I stammered more" absurd. You might be reading this wondering how anyone could possibly desire stammering? We hope this book will open your eyes to the many reasons why.

In addition to society's stereotypes and prejudices, our frustration as stammerers and professionals working in the field of stammering has as much to do with the beliefs of the professionals aiming to support people who stammer. Speech and language therapists can hold the same views as the rest of society, but under the cloak of 'medical expertise'. Stammering is understood in medicine, as in society, as a defect to be 'fixed' or 'overcome'. This medical model perspective attributes difficulties in life caused by impairments (such as visual loss, deafness, or stammering) to defective bodies. Consequently, it has led to the development of many medical and therapeutic approaches to remedy and cure these defects. However, all is not as simple as it appears: the medical model makes the person the problem, creates assumptions about 'normality', and promotes judgements about what society considers 'defective'.

The medical model has led to the development of therapy approaches that aim to correct stammered speech back to fluent norms. Consequently, stammerers often come to believe that fluency is a panacea and the gold standard against which their speech should be judged. Rather than enable stammerers to learn to identify, navigate, and challenge the discrimination that makes their lives difficult, they are taught to capitulate to it by doing everything they can to make their speech fluent. Therapy for young children who stammer sets out to facilitate fluency. For adolescents and adults, typically a 'cure' is no longer deemed possible. Instead, the focus shifts to speech management strategies and encouraging psychological and social adaptation to being a person who stammers. Certainly, some people who stammer have benefited from these interventions. However, at best these attempts put a sticking plaster over the real issue of society's deep-seated insecurities around difference and at worst they can become complicit in further pedalling prejudice.

Even when people who stammer themselves have attempted to develop and drive new understandings of stammering, they have for the most part remained tethered to the medical model. Charles Van Riper and Joseph Sheehan are two notable examples. Both were speech and language therapists who stammered. They used their own experiences of stammering to redefine clinical practice, in particular encouraging the profession to appreciate the nuanced and profound psychological impact stammering can have. Their therapy approaches abandoned the goal of fluency and encouraged people to stammer well. While the psychological depth and breadth of therapy advocated by Van Riper and Sheehan were positive developments, the overriding aims of these approaches still sought to effect change at the level of the individual and not society. This book looks beyond the narrow confines of therapy to structural, attitudinal, and physical barriers present in society affecting people who stammer.

Stammering Pride and Prejudice draws upon a different set of theories and concepts to understand stammering. These come from the disability rights movement in the 1970s, that later became formalized into the social model by Vic Finkelstein and Michael Oliver. In short, these views see the way society is structured as disabling rather than physical impairment itself. The person with a spinal injury who is unable to walk is disabled by the fact there is no ramp access to a building rather than their spinal injury. These ideas, which were so transformative for physical impairments, had passed the stammering community by until the last decade. Yet, as Michael Oliver himself points out in his heartfelt foreword, the social model is as applicable to stammering. It just requires us to think more creatively. People who stammer may not need ramp access; however, we do need a society willing to listen to and respect our stammered voices. We consider this a basic human right.

Stammering – perhaps as usual – has been reluctant to join in the conversation. Indeed, many people who stammer hesitate to identify as 'disabled'. This hesitation can come from a place of misunderstanding and stigma. Disability, as defined by the social model, is a dynamic process, not an inherent characteristic. Therefore, disability is experienced when a person is unable to participate fully in society due to a mismatch between their body and the environment around them. It is not simply a descriptive term for people with significant physical or cognitive impairments, like an inability to walk or a lower IQ. People who stammer may not define themselves as disabled for fear of offending people with more 'significant' disabilities or, more disconcertingly, for fear of becoming associated with people who are often seen as 'broken', 'defective', and 'other' by society. Whether people who stammer consider themselves disabled or not does not stop them from being disabled by society. As long as society views stammered speech as inferior, they will be disabled by societal norms. We ask people who stammer to embrace the socially-constructed concept of disability; we gain strength by aligning ourselves with others who also experience daily barriers, prejudice, and discrimination because their bodies do not meet society's expectations of normality.

The nature of stammering, its variability and hideability, can make it more challenging to understand as disabling. People who stammer are sometimes disabled a lot; sometimes a little. Fluctuations in frequency of stammering may alter how disabled we feel; this may also be altered by the perceived and actual hostility of the speaking environment. A person who chooses silence because of fear of stigma, one who is silenced by their effortful blocks, and one who speaks but is ignored through prejudice are all disabled, albeit in different ways.

Prejudice

Our society is dominated by the story, or narrative, of smooth-talking fluency as the preferred way to speak. Newscasters, politicians, actors are universally fluent. Job vacancies ask for excellent communication and voice-automated systems are unable to understand stammering. Fluency as the 'right' way to speak; stammering as the 'wrong' way to speak is the dominant narrative of our society. This is powerful. These narratives become blueprints for all stories and, as such, the vehicles through which we come to understand the stories of others and ourselves. Knowingly or unknowingly, we adopt the narratives that are familiar to us, thereby replicating the master societal story.

People who stammer are conditioned by society to think it is ugly to stammer and therefore often share this point of view too. Wendell Johnson famously defined stammering as what we do trying not to stammer. While a bit of a tautology, the definition has proven useful for describing the wide range of behaviours we use to avoid stammering. However, little attention has been given to why we are ubiquitously trying not to stammer. Our stammering may make speech effortful and it can be unsettling to experience its loss of control. But these experiences do not justify the wide-ranging avoidance strategies we often use to escape moments of stammering and the lengths to which we sometimes go to pass as fluent.

In the past, our inclination to hide stammering has been framed as a personal failing: we are socially anxious, timid, or just too weak to be open about who we are. The truth is, we often try not to stammer for good reasons. We are punished for stammering; it goes against the dominant societal narrative. We experience teasing and bullying as children and discrimination and prejudice as adults. As some of the authors document, even society's best attempts at helping us when we are young can further this prejudice. Therapy can reinforce that stammering is not a legitimate way of speaking and that if we want to be taken seriously we must try to be fluent. We are taught from a young age, by the adults whom we trust, that fluent speech is more valuable than stammered speech.

Prejudice takes many forms. It can be blatant, but it can also be subtle, just part of the landscape. Discrimination can occur in the absence of outright attacks on us and our speech. These instances occur when we are simply not considered and our experiences of speaking are ignored. When it is assumed that everyone is or should be fluent, we suffer. The authors in this book explore their own experiences of prejudice. They highlight the abundant evidence that people who stammer are discriminated against and stigmatized. They also describe how this societal stigma changes our understanding of stammering from a natural variation in speech production to a clinical defect with many negative consequences.

Pride

Whilst stammerers have been repeating the tropes of the 20th century, the conversation in disability has exploded into the 21st. In particular, we have seen the emergence of movements, such as neurodiversity, that re-imagine the concept of underlying 'impairment', or a 'weakened body', from disability. 'Impairments' are seen as natural variation and an intrinsic part of the rich diversity of humanity. If we set up society to support these variations, then we can all benefit from them: Tourette's brings vocal spontaneity, autism increased attention to detail, and dyslexia creative writing. In tandem, disabled people are beginning to draw positive and empowering identities from their disabled experience. This thinking has not developed in a vacuum. In a wider context, these positive ways of conceptualizing disability increasingly intersect, overlap, and draw from activism in other areas of society, like womens, LGBTQI+, black and ethnic minority rights movements, and more. We live in a society that is beginning to understand that difference is not defect.

The dawn of stammering or dysfluency pride, chronicled in this book, shows the beginnings of a similar movement among the stammering community. This takes a different view of research findings into the cause of stammering. It sees the gene changes that predispose to stammering as natural human variation, not damaging mutations; and the neurological changes people who stammer have as differences rather than abnormalities in brain wiring.

It questions who has the right to decide whether the way of speaking these natural genetic and neurological differences lead to is inferior to fluent speech. Biologically, stammering comprises a plethora of unique speech patterns; it is only when placed in a certain social context that it becomes a disorder. We can each choose how to define stammering. We can accept the dominant definition of our society or we can choose to define it as a unique and valuable way of speaking.

Stammering pride is a counter narrative to the dominant societal narrative around fluency. We open the book with a transcript of Erin Schick's performance poem 'Honest Speech'. Her open, direct resistance to social norms and reframing of stammering as her voice's 'greatest symphony' and 'the most honest part of me' encapsulates the growing movement of stammering pride. A counter narrative only makes sense in relation to what it is countering. The term identifies it as a positional category, in tension with another category. Thus, stammering pride can only be fully understood in relation to prejudice. Stammering pride asks individuals to question the discriminatory fluent norms and ableist attitudes of society and take a much more empowering view of their speech. Like Erin's poem, it invites us to resist these current fluent values, to stammer loudly and proudly, and show society what we sound like.

Counter narratives take different forms in this book. Through literature, theorising, research, art, photography and poetry, experiences of stammering which often remain invisible, unnamed and unacknowledged in mainstream society are brought into focus. Many of these narratives are deeply reflective, infusing personal history and experience with new meaning, complexity and depth. As a reader, expect to be challenged, unsettled, and moved. The different chapters in this book explore questions of inclusion and exclusion, the social construction of normalcy, and the profound effects of social and communication norms and expectations. It also looks into the boundaries and interactions between the individual who stammers and the collective, between the self and society. Many of these narratives uphold the value of breaking away from socially conceived norms and harnessing the unique experience of stammering in its own right.

As stammering is reclaimed as a different, legitimate, and valuable means of communication, a radical conversation around stammering gain emerges. Arguably, until we have a reason to stammer, until we choose to stammer freely and openly because it benefits us, stammering will remain positioned as the negative opposite of fluency. Other people will not value our stammering if we cannot value it ourselves. Pride denotes a feeling of deep pleasure or satisfaction derived from our own achievements, or from qualities or possessions that are widely admired. Stammering pride demands recognition for what the stammered voice adds to conversations, interactions, roles and relationships - not for what it lacks.

A number of chapters in this book demonstrate how stammering renders simple verbal exchanges anything but trite. Stammering brings novelty, unpredictability, and excitement. In the silence of stammering is the potential of what is yet to come. The unexpectedness of stammering forces both listener and speaker into a space of vulnerability, which can make everyday conversations immediately intimate and sincere. Thus, stammering can create opportunities, open doors to relationships, and foster a depth of connection that has benefit for the person who stammers and for society. The two-way nature of interaction creates an opportunity for every listener to meet the openness and authenticity of stammering in a way that fosters shared respect and intimacy.

What is dominant and what is subjugated in our society is fluid. This will become apparent as you try to understand where the contributors position themselves in the stories that they tell as they navigate the 'inside/outside' dynamics of society. What emerges are the multiple layers of positioning and the complexity in this negotiation. All the personal narratives in this book highlight the important influence of the dominant cultural scripts on their lives. What is powerful about the stories presented here is that they expand the boundaries of these dominant cultural storylines by offering alternative narratives around stammering that can be told. Each of the narratives offers a personal example of making sense of and moving beyond stereotypical conceptualizations of stammering as defective or a disorder to be treated. This is liberating, not just for the contributors who both author and live the story of their lives, but for the reader and for society at large as we too are unshackled from conforming to dominant and self-limiting narratives. It is an invitation to us all to explore and value our own uniqueness in this world.

Stammering Pride and Prejudice

The title of this book reflects its contents. We borrowed the Jane Austen pun from a conference held in 2016 at City Lit, London, exploring stammering from a social model perspective. To begin with, it was a working title, a place-holder, for when something more original came along. But, while other things have changed from inception to print – Chris alone got married, finished a PhD, and became an assistant Professor – the title has not. It succinctly captures what this book is about: the current prejudice and stigma surrounding stammering in society counterpoised by the pride and rich meanings people who stammer are beginning to take in their speech.

Stammering: Pride and Prejudice comprises an eclectic mix of personal essays, art, and poetry related to stammering. Each piece is unique and can be read individually. We placed them in an order that begins in the depths of prejudice, wanders through therapy, and arrives at pride. We encourage you, however, to dip in and out of the book as you wish. The book draws on disability theory to create a multidimensional understanding of stammering in today's society. But academic thought alone does not bring about change. For these ideas to be of real worth, they must benefit people in their day-to-day, messy and difficult lives. *Stammering Pride and Prejudice* is filled with stories and experiences of people who stammer grappling with these ideas. Some of these are empowering, some bitter, some celebratory, some joyful. Others are more practical, personal accounts about how the social model can drive cultural change, for the benefit of both people who stammer and wider society.

Academic texts can become weighed down with jargon and innumerable references, particularly to readers unfamiliar to the subject. We have tried to avoid this and make the book accessible to those unacquainted with the language of disability studies and academia. We decided against a formal reference style, instead opting to integrate references into the writing, and asked authors to limit their bibliographies. We valued the unique voices of our authors. Accordingly their literary style has been maintained, and choice of 'stammerer', 'stutterer', or 'person who stammers/stutters' respected.

We found art central to our message. Art allows us to see, hear, feel, and think about stammering differently. Art can identify, challenge, and alter the connotations that accompany our everyday language. Visual art can accomplish this by doing away with language altogether. A picture is worth a thousand words, precisely because it does not use any. Language-based art, such as poetry and prose, still use language, but in new and exciting ways. We hope the artwork we have included will help highlight our prejudices and biases and in doing so manage to free our words and thinking from their historical chains.

Final thoughts

If you are the type of person who reads the final lines of a book before buying it, we want to draw your attention to a borrowed line from Chris' final chapter. He quotes from Walt Whitman's poem 'Song of Myself':

'Do I contradict myself?
Very well then I contradict myself,
(I am large, I contain multitudes.)'

Stammering can be understood in a multitude of ways. We wanted *Stammering Pride and Prejudice* to make the sentence "I am learning to stammer more" a little less absurd. To give people a more nuanced and positive way to understand their stammering. This does not mean that stammering is always a garden of roses. It can be a curse, a nuisance, and a gift all at the same time. The diverse voices in this book reflect this. They contradict each other and, sometimes, even themselves; they are likely to contradict your own thinking on stammering too. We invite you, however, to resist the temptation to try to resolve any differences prematurely, defensively, or artificially. Rather, to sit with the tensions, divisions and the contradictions painted by the book's more coherent and complete picture of people's experience.

Honest speech

Erin Schick

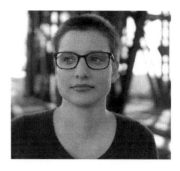

This photo was taken on the Steel Bridge over the Willamette River in Portland, where I lived when I wrote this poem.

The barn owl communicates with its mates and offspring using a complex system of hissing, screeching, squawking, and facial muscle manipulation
Survival is dependent upon creating a voice so unique it can be recognized by loved ones in an instant

I argue, the cause of my ssstutter is not neurologic
It's got to be something dd-eeper
Something dd-esperate to –be remembered

My mouth spit-shines syllables 'till they sss-parkle
'Till my voice is the only one like it
This is nnnot a speech imm—pediment
My voice is an instrument
My ss-tutter its greatest symphony
My speech com-pposed by God
I buy –tth-ree –ggrapefuit and I –sstutter
I –sstudy –ssociology and I —-sstutter
I like tzatz-tza-tz-taztziki and I –sstutter
The stattacctto of repetition is an unpre—ddictable –pp-recussion
The struggle for every syllable a reminder that I have not always had this voice
This –stage, a gift of spotlights

It seems there is a new kind of privilege here
In being understood the first time
In breath, calm and measured stripping speech of nuance
In passing-as-fluent to spare someone else embarrassment
For too long I have been afraid of my own name

The word invented only to -d—esscribe me
I have let it sit heavy in my ttthroat
A tool of b-betrayal
I introduce myself and I ssstutter
I'm a –poet and I –ssttutter
I call my –-pparents, and I –ssttutter
I love you and I stutter
I love myssself and I ssstutter

The sstuttering is the most honest part of me
It is the only thing that never lies
It is how I know I still have a voice
I am still -being heard
I am still here
When I stutter I am speaking my own language fluently
When I sound like this I know my loved ones can find me
This is what I sssound like when I speak for myself
This is what I sound like
This is what I sound like.

An introduction to stuttering and disability theory: Misfits in meaning

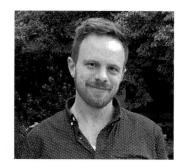

Joshua St. Pierre

Introduction

I have stuttered since I can remember and my unsteady speech has, until recently, been a source of deep shame that I have tried to eliminate. I have felt deep shame not only about how I spoke but also of myself. Like many people who stutter, I have spent countless hours in speech therapy in the effort to sound and be included as 'normal'. It was only when I stumbled upon disability studies in grad school that I realized my understanding of stuttering was far too narrow. I in fact had the problem backwards: what if my way of communicating is interpreted as abnormal by others because it conflicts with a particular set of values and social structures? What if I don't need to change? It is hard to overstate the empowering and revolutionary truth of this simple claim.

In this chapter I outline three models of disability in relation to stuttering: the medical model, the social model, and the political/relational model. A 'model' of disability is a framework through which society understands and manages the concept of disability (Withers, 2012). There are many more models than those discussed here.[1] However, the medical, social, and political/relational models offer a concise picture of how our society and culture currently understands stuttering and how we might reimagine stuttering differently.

The medical model of disability

When most people think about disability today, they are using the language and framework of the medical model of disability. Who dares dispute the idea that disability is a biological problem of individual bodies? However, all ideas have a history, and looking carefully at the medical model can help us ask better questions about disability and respond to it more thoughtfully. A.J. Withers, a Canadian disability activist, offers a concise definition of the medical model that I will detail below:

> "A clinical approach to disability which focuses on the use of diagnostic tools to identify pathology and make interventions in that pathology in order to cure or minimize it. Under this framework, disability is based in the body, normal is constructed as ideal, disabled people are dependent, and our identities are tragedies in need of intervention" (2012, p.31).

The medical model can be a helpful way to understand disability in certain contexts, but it is not the *only* way. The medical model, moreover, has built-in goals of eliminating and curing disability which tend to be taken for granted but, as I will argue, have dangerous effects. My concern is thus with neither medicine nor science in themselves, but the way they are *used* and their authority over increasingly more aspects of our lives. Allow me to fill out this definition by examining four points from Withers' quotation in greater detail.

First, the medical model confines disability to **individual bodies**. Take a brief contrast. In the religious model, disability does not reside in the individual per se but is rather a *sign* of something larger like divine intervention, divine order, or sin. Disability is of course always embodied by individual people, but there is nothing like genetics rooting its presence in the individual body itself. On the other hand, the medical model (which originates in the late-18th century) is thoroughly scientific in its understanding of and approach to the world. In the realm of the medical model, the source or truth of disability (what it *really is*) can only be decided by scientific observation, calculation, measurement, and empirical facts. Under this 'medical gaze' that systematically excludes religious folk, and (as I will argue below) political explanations of disability, disability becomes a fixed characteristic of individual biological bodies. It *is* deviant anatomy; it *is* abnormal development. This framework offers no other option.

Second, the medical model divides the wide array of human variation into two categories: **normal** and **abnormal** (i.e., pathological). This distinction underlies the life sciences and the medical model's expert authority over disability. What is this distinction? In one sense, 'normal' simply refers to a statistical point on a bell curve that describes species-typical characteristics. It is true, for example, that human beings are *typically* bipedal, over four feet tall, and possess only two copies of chromosome #21. But the idea of normalcy is more complex than a mathematical average, since when medical experts make definitive claims about which human characteristics are normal or pathological based on their scientific expertise, they are always doing two implicit things: marking a hierarchy and expressing social value judgements. To take a mundane example, both red hair and stuttering stem from genetic mutations that occur in roughly 1% of the population. Both phenotypes are statistically atypical yet only the latter shows up on medicine's radar as abnormal or pathological. I happen to both stutter and have red hair, but have never heard anyone discuss the 'risk' of my future children inheriting the latter. This is because 'abnormal' is not simply mathematical but always marks a hierarchy –a particularly *undesirable* deviation. Yet we must ask: who decides what forms of human variation are desirable, undesirable, or neutral? Is this the realm of medicine?

Psychiatric diagnosis offers an even more clear example of the way that 'normalcy' is not objective but expresses social value judgements. When the American Psychiatric Association introduced the *Diagnostic and Statistical Manual of Mental Disorders* (or DSM-I) in 1952, it contained diagnoses for 106 abnormal psychiatric conditions. When the DSM-5 was released in 2013, it contained over 300 diagnoses. More significant than the sheer number of abnormal conditions that pop in and out of existence is the fact that psychiatry reflects social values. For example, the DSM-I and II classified homosexuality as a sexual deviation and was not removed until the publication of the DSM-III in 1973. Disability is a category of deviance which is not neutral but politically loaded. Medicine considers individuals or groups to be abnormal (and thus within the medical domain) that society has already decided are unwanted or morally wrong. When society's opinion changes, medical intervention is often no longer considered appropriate. Medicine thus both reflects social stigmas and helps create them.

Normalcy in this fuller sense describes what a society desires and aspires towards – normalcy is an ideal. It is at once a scientific *and* a cultural categorization, an objective description of the body/mind and a projection of what a body/mind *should* be. This is why when 'abnormalities' are discovered during a prenatal ultrasound the 'objective facts' are typically explained in a voice flooded with tragedy. How could it be any other way? This model rests on a hierarchy that equates normal with 'health' or 'wellbeing' and disability with suffering. Disability is always framed as negative, understood to be a drain on society that destroys, among other things, the quality of life for families and individuals (Kafer, 2013). In short: disability as pathology marks a tragic deviation from an ideal life trajectory.

Third, the medical model is **clinical** in nature and stakes its expert claim to the truth of disability in scientific knowledge. Diagnostic tools give medical professionals seemingly objective knowledge about the body that patients cannot access. On the basis of this knowledge and through the clinical *relationship*, medical professionals become expert authorities on disability that disabled people defer to for their own wellbeing. Disabled people, put otherwise, are transformed into pathologized recipients of treatment who (in order to access treatment) must recognize themselves in medicalized terms. For example, in the first edition of *Speech Correction: Principles and Methods* (1963), Charles Van Riper describes this recognition as the 'objective attitude': the "unemotional admission of [one's] speech difference as a problem to be solved" (p.362). To have disabled people accept the terms of the medical model welds them to expert knowledge and authority. This asymmetrical relation is often marginalizing since, as Withers states, "our own experiences can be disregarded or understood to be false if they contradict medical opinion" (p.35). Recent moves towards 'patient-centred' therapy in SLP (DiLollo & Favreau, 2010; Luterman, 2016) that seek more balance of authority in the clinical relationship are certainly welcome as they lower the intensity of the relationship, but even here the fundamental structure of expert and patient remains. In contrast, I argue that people who stutter should have control over not just the type of therapy we receive, but the terms that frame the entire discussion. *Is* stuttering a pathology? What *should* the role of expert intervention be? As long as Medicine is the stage for policy, research, and funding debates in/about the stuttering community, our knowledge and desires as disabled people can only be marginalized.[2]

Fourth, it follows that within the medical model, disability as pathology is a problem to be solved through expert **intervention**. As I have argued, the medical model creates expert authorities who define disability as a problem that only they can fix. Since the medical model imagines disability as simultaneously an individual biological breakdown, as tragic suffering, and as a threat to the functioning of society, expert intervention to 'fix' individual bodies is always deemed necessary. This automatic impulse to cure and rehabilitate makes it nearly impossible to comprehend disability as something that does not require expert intervention. While other models (like the religious and charity) also frame intervention in terms of tragedy, the medical model has adopted this framework by grounding it in the scientific truth of the disabled body. It is this scientific claim over the truth of disability that provides the strong momentum for intervention in our society.

Having considered the four pillars of the medical model it is worth asking directly how this model applies to stuttering. Since discussions within the stuttering community have been dominated by the medical model (and, to a lesser degree, the charity model), this is an easy answer. The medical model defines stuttering as a distinctly biological problem rooted in both genetics and neurology (with secondary causes afforded to psychology) and takes this definition to be an objective fact. Jackson, Quesal and Yaruss (2012), for example, offer an exemplary medicalized definition of stuttering:

> "Stuttering is a neurobiological lack of integration of the underlying processes of planning and producing language and speech that, upon verbal execution, can lead to interruptions in the acoustic speech signal (e.g., blocks, part-word repetitions, disfluencies) and physical struggle (e.g., tension). These surface behaviors may not be present, however, when the speaker exhibits communicative avoidance (e.g., circumlocutions, fillers). The underlying features may lead to surface behaviors, *as well as* emotional and cognitive reactions. Depending on the individual, these may result in significant difficulties in communication and an adverse impact on the speaker's quality of life. The physical symptoms, emotional and cognitive reactions, and impact on the speaker's life all comprise the disorder of stuttering."
> [emphasis in original]

Stuttering is here notably a *lack* that is rooted in biology. The secondary features of stuttering like communication avoidance and quality of life can all trace back not to structural issues in society but to the abnormality of the stuttering body. It is likely, as I explain in the next section, that most SLPs likely do not think in terms of the 'medical model' since they often use a hybrid model somewhere in between the medical and social: the International Classification of Functioning, Disability, and Health (ICF) that was established by the World Health Organization. While this model does attempt to capture the complex experience of disability, I will argue that it remains fundamentally rooted in a medicalized understanding of the world.

In sum, a central concern with the medical model's grounding in pathologization and intervention is that it can often reinforce the oppression of disabled people. As Withers explains, the medical model's primary function is "to change oppressed individuals but leave the social structures that enable oppression intact" (p.34). This of course makes sense from the medical perspective: if disability is an individual pathology, then changing building codes, architecture, laws, social attitudes, cultural representation, etc., address the *effects* of disability but not disability itself. The medical model moves past symptoms to reach the 'real' cause or source of disability. Similarly, SLPs are rightly concerned with the quality of life of their clients. But, as I will argue below, if disability is primarily a social and political rather than biological matter, then seeking medical/therapeutic solutions is a profound misdiagnosis that in many ways only increases the stigma and oppression that disabled people face.

The social model of disability

The social model of disability was born in the UK during the 1970s. The main idea behind this model is the distinction between 'impairment' and 'disability'– where impairment is a medical condition but disability a social condition. As the Union of the Physically Impaired Against Segregation (UPIAS; an early UK disability rights group) stated: "In our view it is society which disables physically impaired people. Disability is something imposed on top of our impairments by the way we are unnecessarily isolated and excluded from full participation in society" (1976; quoted in Oliver, 1996, p.22). If impairment is congenital blindness, disability is not having a lease agreement available in a screen-reader format. If impairment is paraplegia, disability is experienced when a flight of stairs blocks access to a building. The blind person and wheelchair user are disabled in this model by such barriers. The central point here is that 'disability' is no longer an individual or personal issue but the result of how society organizes in ways that exclude people with impairments. Impaired bodies are disabled by society.

The main political strategy of the social model is accordingly to remove social barriers that impede disabled people both from full participation in the workforce and society and from exercising control over their lives. Disability activists and theorists describe this strategy using the metaphor of 'access'. The response to a world of barriers that disable people is not to remove impairment but to make the world *itself* more accessible. Creating access involves, for example, removing stigma about disability, providing closed captions and ASL interpretation, making public transportation usable for a wide variety of bodies, or providing support for independent living. This is useful since many disabled people *can't* be medically cured (or rehabilitated) and are often exhausted by costly and time-consuming therapies they wouldn't need if their world were easier to navigate.

From a historical perspective, the social model was extremely important in reframing how disabled people conceived themselves. Defining disability in the language of civil rights allowed disabled people to think of themselves (for the first time) as a social group bound by a shared oppression. Naming something is important, and we could now talk of 'ableism' – the systemic discrimination in favour of able-bodied people – similar to racism or sexism. This shift was profoundly empowering, as activist and writer Liz Crow explains:

> "For years now this social model of disability has enabled me to confront, survive and even surmount countless situations of exclusion and discrimination... It has played a central role in promoting disabled people's individual self-worth, collective identity and political organization. I don't think it is an exaggeration to say that the social model has saved lives" (1996, p.207; cited in Withers, 2012, p.87).

When disability is understood first and foremost not as an individual but a collective experience and identity, then Deaf, blind, quadriplegic, and Autistic people (for example) could start to organize politically and fight *as a group* for equality and justice.[3] Tom Shakespeare and Nicholas Watson, two UK disability theorists and activists, put it this way: "Suddenly, people were able to understand that they weren't at fault: society was. They didn't need to change: society needed to change" (2001, p.11).

How, then, does stuttering fit into this model? Our impairment is the fact that we speak with hesitations, blocks, prolongations, and repetitions due to specific neurological and genetic factors. We are disabled, on the other hand, by the fast pace of society; by people who interrupt our speech; by those who deny us jobs because of our speech; and by a multitude of ableist stereotypes, biases and stigmas. People with communication impairments are not excluded from social and economic participation by physical barriers such as stairs and broken elevators but by more abstract barriers like how society organizes time and practises communication. The disability rights movement has historically focused on physical barriers to access which has excluded from proper consideration disabilities like stuttering. Commenting on this lack, Judy Duchan (an SLP and historian of SLP) has argued for a broadening of the notion of access to include 'communication access'. As she writes:

"Such attention [to communication access] would require these historians [of disability] to broaden their interpretation of 'equal access' to include depictions of language, literacy, and conceptual barriers. And the access 'destinations' would be related to communication and social participation, as well as places. A history of communication access might, for example, focus on language, literacy, or social barriers that must be overcome to achieve an 'appropriate education' or a 'reasonable accommodation' or a 'least restrictive environment'" (2006, para. 8).

Thinking with Duchan, creating access for stutterers could mean offering extended speaking times and alternate forms of participation not just in the classroom (an accommodation included in most education plans for stutterers) but the boardroom, the checkout line, and general society. It could mean actually enforcing existing anti-discrimination legislation.

The social model represents an important moment in the history of disability activism, yet it is not the end of the conversation. Three critiques of this model stand out in particular. First, the social model's stance against medicalization is somewhat halfhearted since medical abnormalities still exist in the form of 'impairment' but are simply not the focus of intervention. That is, we should recognize that what the medical model terms 'disability' the social model essentially re-labels as 'impairment'. To cite the UPIAS again, impairment means: "lacking all or part of a limb, or having a defective limb, organism or mechanism of the body". The social model drives a wedge between the biological and the social, which allows activists to claim 'disability' as a political identity that is distinct from impairment. The problem with this move is that it also leaves entirely unchallenged Medicine's authority over the *impaired* body. One can only be considered disabled and receive the necessary accommodations if one is first categorized and recognized as impaired. In addition, being anchored to the medical model limits the range and effectiveness of disability activism. The social model (and activists working within this framework) cannot escape the orbit of the medical model and must ultimately accept and work within its descriptions of and authority over the body.

Second, the claim that 'we are disabled by society' leaves out personal aspects of disability like physical pain, chronic illness and fatigue. The social model's focus on external barriers is important, but as Liz Crow states: "Many people find that it is their experience of their bodies – and not only disabling barriers such as inaccessible public transport – which make political involvement difficult.

For example, an individual's capacity to attend meetings and events might be restricted because of limited energy" (1996, p.210). Similarly, people who stutter are disabled not only by society but also by the physical pain and frustration of trying to push out words. Even in a perfect world without discrimination stuttering bodies would cause discomfort. How can we account for the complex relationship we have with our bodies?

Third, and directly related, the social model understands disability to be inherently negative. When 'disability' is defined as a form of oppression burdened on impairment (which as a medical category is itself negative and tragic) it becomes difficult to imagine disability as something positive that we might genuinely desire. As Liz Crow states above, the social model has played a central role in providing disabled people with self-worth, but the firm distinction between impairment/disability can, I believe, obstruct the more radical possibilities of disability activism.

Before turning to the political/relational model, it is worth noting that Speech-Language Pathology uses a model somewhere in between the medical and social. In 2001, the World Health Organization endorsed the International Classification of Functioning, Disability, and Health (ICF). The framework takes into consideration not only the body but its environment. Disability describes how certain 'bodily structures' and 'bodily functions' interact with the environment to restrict and make possible 'activities' and 'participation' in the world. SLPs such as J. Scott Yaruss and Robert Quesal (2004) have eagerly applied the ICF model to stuttering since the model aims at a holistic picture of 'health' and can thus account for much of the complexity of a communication disability. Yet the limitation of models (or more accurately, systems of classification) like the ICF is that they are purely 'descriptive', which means they make no claim on what society *should* be like, *whether* pharmaceutical companies should be intimately involved in our lives, or *why* slow speech impedes participation in the world. It cannot account for political structures of ableism and provides little motivation or way forward to change the world and make it more just. In short, classification models like ICF can provide more detailed and contextual assessments of stuttering which can in turn provide 'better' treatment, but unlike the social model it does not attempt to challenge the authority of the medical model.

The political/relational model of disability

Since the social model is part of an ongoing conversation in disability studies, the critiques of the social model have produced both updated versions of this model (e.g., Shakespeare, 2006) as well as new models that build on and try to think beyond the impairment/disability distinction. In this section I focus on what Kafer has termed the 'political/relational' model, yet it is worth noting that this model overlaps in many ways with what Withers terms the 'radical model' of disability (pp.81-97) and what David Mitchell and Sharon Snyder (2005) call the 'cultural model'. As an initial point of reference, one could say that if disability is a cosmic *sign* in the religious model, a biological *pathology* in the medical model, a social *oppression* in the social model, then it is a political *relation* in the aptly named political/relational model. This requires some unpacking.

As I argued above, one of the pillars of the medical model is the belief that human characteristics divide into two categories: normal and pathological. The political/relational model challenges this idea at a fundamental level. Ron Amundson is a philosopher of biology who has forcefully argued that "the concept of normality is a biological error" (2000, p.34): that normality and abnormality do not reflect biological reality. Rather, what we find in the world is a rich tapestry of biological *variation* that cannot fit into these narrow medical categories. Amundson's full argument is obviously more complex (hinging on the importance of 'developmental plasticity'), but the upshot for Amundson and disability theorists who follow this line of thought is that arranging the complex world of biological diversity into two categories is anything but objective. Normalcy and abnormalcy are distinctly *political* categories used to sort human differences according to which forms of biological variation we as a society find acceptable and useful in our specific historical context. Understanding disability to be first and foremost a political rather than biological category opens a lot of space to rethink disability and contest the meanings and categories that are attached to our lives.

The 'neurodiversity' moment that has become prominent within Autistic self-advocacy circles speaks to this important shift towards understanding disability as an expression of biological variation. Nick Walker (an Autistic author and scholar) describes an "infinite variation in neurocognitive functioning within our species" such that: "The idea that there is one 'normal' or 'healthy' type of brain or mind, or one 'right' style of neurocognitive functioning, is a culturally constructed fiction, no more valid (and no more conducive to a healthy society or to the overall well-being of humanity) than the idea that there is one 'normal' or 'right' ethnicity, gender, or culture" (2014).

As the comedian and disability activist Nina G has argued, stuttering fits well into the neurodiversity paradigm (Stuttertalk, p.563). Scientific research has revealed a neurological basis for stuttering, but such research is always framed by the language of normalcy. Yet it is only a small (though significant) step to think about the neurological basis of stuttering in terms of neurological diversity rather than abnormality. This is the direction Cristóbal Loriente (2009) takes in his theory of 'transfluency' in which "The speaker's speech pattern (whether fluent, cluttered or stuttering) just exists, and there are as many speech patterns as individuals. Just as different sexual orientations and expressions of diversity such as left-handedness are not considered to be inherently pathological, no particular speech pattern is considered to be pathological" (p.139). Dysfluent speech expresses a difference, not a deviance, and re-defining stuttering in non-medicalized terms is essential for stuttering activism to carve a place for dysfluent voices in the world. Redefining stuttering is needed to reclaim authority over our dysfluent bodies, to *reimagine* what stuttering could be, and thus to speak on our own terms.

The argument that stuttering is a form of biological diversity requires consideration of the relational character of disability. Kafer (2013) argues that disability is always experienced in and through relationships. At one level, this means simply that disability always exists in a social context. Discriminatory prejudices, stigmas and practices always travel through relationships with family, friends, co-workers, medical professionals, etc. The meaning of disability never occurs in isolation: this is especially true with a communication disability such as stuttering. The deeper point, however, is that when we talk of structural issues like physical, economic and social barriers we are still describing relations. Within the social model, disability is experienced through barriers like a flight of stairs that blocks access to a building or a public transit system without the tactile and audio cues required by blind people for access. The political/relational model highlights the fact that architecture is never simply concrete and steel but a complex *relation* between people and their environments. Who do we design our material environments for? What types of bodies can inhabit public spaces? Who is permitted and expected to occupy our social environment and who is not? And, most importantly, *why* have we arranged our world in this way?

I've thus come to understand disability, reading disability theorist Rosemarie Garland-Thomson, as a mismatch between bodies and their environments: an attempt to fit a square peg into a round hole. Our society designs the world to fit 'normal' bodies with little thought to how this excludes many others such that those who misfit fall into categories such as 'disabled'. Disability occurs when a body enters an environment that does not support its form or function (Garland–Thomson, 2011, p.594). For example, automated telephone menus are not designed for my stuttered voice. Neither do workplace expectations of clear communication nor conversational turn-taking customs accommodate the hesitations in my speech. The society we encounter is designed for fluent speakers and gives little thought to how this excludes those of us who stutter. This misfit between how we talk and how society *demands* that we talk exposes and makes us vulnerable to ableist social discrimination. The vulnerability comes neither from our bodies (the medical model) nor strictly speaking the environment (the social model) but the misfitting relation between these two realities.

To put the two pieces of the political/relational model together, stuttering can therefore be understood as a political category applied to *certain* neurodiverse and dysfluent bodies that describes not a biological truth of the body but a relationship between people and their social and communicative environments. To speak dysfluently is to speak more slowly than our society allows. It is to stretch, repeat, and block on words. But this, in itself, is no pathology. When dysfluency is transformed into a pathology called 'stuttering', this tells us less about our bodies in themselves than it does about the relation between the social world and our bodies – what speech patterns our society finds acceptable and useful. It is of course true that stuttering has been an object of fascination throughout much of Western history (see Bobrick, 1995). Stuttering is, as Marcel Wingate (1997) says, a "curious disorder" that many physicians have poked at throughout the centuries. Yet it is important to note that stuttering was pathologized and first defined as a *social problem* during the late-19th and early-20th centuries – right when industrialized and democratic societies were gaining speed and began requiring fluent speech to operate efficiently (St. Pierre & St. Pierre, 2018). The need for a world of smooth speech created a large misfit with dysfluent bodies. The definition and meaning of a speech 'impediment' thus always shifts in relation to economic and social contexts. In a society largely made up of farmers and labourers, what counts as a speech impediment will be much different than in a modern social environment saturated with information and organized around communication. On the flip-side, what counts as normal speech is now a shrinking target as speech experts within the medical model find ever-more precise forms of speech difference to classify as deviant.

Just as fixing individual bodies misses the point, so does seeking to 'change society' – as if we ourselves are not part of society. The goal for the political/relational model, rather, is to transform how dysfluent people and able-bodied people relate, to transform the relation of authority between people who stutter and medical experts (such as SLPs), and to transform the relation that stutterers have to themselves. This strategy seeks to transform our relations and thus change society *and* ourselves at the same time. This is much more than a change of attitude, seeking acceptance, or even removing barriers to participation. It is a radical transformation of the value of diversity and the place for disability or dysfluency in the world. To fill this out, allow me to return to the three critiques of the social model I raised above.

First, the political/relational model challenges the expertise of medical professionals over disabled lives and highlights the importance of reclaiming the terms of the discussion. The motto 'nothing about us without us' used widely in disability activist communities is summarized by James Charlton (1998) as the proclamation that disabled people "know what is best for themselves and their community" (p.4). This means, for example, that debates about policy should involve disabled people - those actually affected by said policy. Or again, researchers should take their cues from disabled people when deciding what issues are most pressing and should be held accountable to these communities for their research and the effects of their research. Even though the medical model regularly discredits the experience of disabled people, disabled people are nevertheless the experts on their lives. 'Nothing about us without us' pre-dates the political/relational model, popularized by the disability community in the 1990s during the heyday of the social model. However, the idea behind this proclamation arguably gains even more power when it can apply - using the social model's terms - to impairment as well as to disability. That is to say, because disability is a political matter before a biological one, the political/relational model refuses to concede that medical experts hold the truth about stuttering. Stuttering is not a pathology but a form of variation that has been squeezed into medical categories. Reclaiming authority over dysfluency means defining it (and ourselves) on our own terms and seeking medical intervention on our own terms.

This last point deserves additional attention since it is easy to imagine the political/relational as a rejection of medical intervention. I see a doctor regularly and expect her medical knowledge to be up-to-date. Medicine plays an important role in our lives. It is important to make room for people who want to change their bodies in response to ableism and/or disability. Many people will want to seek therapy to change their stutter or to minimize the physical pain of stuttering. This is both acceptable and welcome. Recognizing that the medical model is always political simply allows us to ask better questions about intervention and to seek intervention on our own terms. Who has access to care? For how long? Do they have choices? A community of people who stutter needs to be able to decide for ourselves what role speech therapy gets to have in our lives, and that will not happen when the discussion is dominated by the language and terminology of SLP and when experts continue to define our voices for us.

Second, while the firm distinction between impairment and disability leaves out physical aspects of stuttering such as pain and discomfort, the political/relational model of disability acknowledges and makes space for these realities. It is quite possible to value disability as a form of human variation but also remain honest about the challenges of living in/as a body. Our bodies are not always pleasant places to live. However, it is important to recognize that ageing and pain are not restricted to 'disabled bodies' and need not be considered a defect. That is to say, the limitations and frustrations of inhabiting a body is a reality for *all* bodies, not just those labelled pathological. Limitation is what it means to live as a body! While disability "gives even greater urgency to the fears and limitations associated with the body" (Siebers, 2013, p.284) the answer is neither to shrug off the body nor place the blame on disability. Thinking about embodiment in this way allows us to appreciate our voices and unique patterns of speech while recognizing *through a critical lens* the challenges our voices and bodies can present.

Third, when disability itself is understood not as a social oppression but as a form of human variation that fits and misfit with the environment, it becomes easier to imagine disability positively. Stigma and negative stereotypes about disability contribute in significant ways to the oppression that disabled people face. Negative views of disability exist 'out there' in the world but are also internalized by disabled people such that we begin to believe the stigmas and stereotypes told about us. Something stronger than 'acceptance' is needed to root out internalized ableism, and claiming 'disability pride' can go a long way in combating ableism in all its forms. Withers writes that "Disabled people are not problems; we are diverse and offer important understandings of the world that should be celebrated rather than marginalized" (p.98). Dysfluency likewise offers an important perspective and critique of our fluent world. Why *should* people have to speak fluently to be taken seriously? Why *does* our modern world move at such a breakneck speed? Is there a different way to think about communication? Why shouldn't we love the sound and unpredictability of the speech patterns that are uniquely our own? Dysfluency – a form of human variation; a different way of living in the world – is something we can genuinely desire. It demands a rethinking of our relationships with one another; it requires that we listen more carefully to each other; that we slow down. To be at home in dysfluent bodies requires that we begin to make a habitable world for dysfluency. Dysfluency requires community to flourish.

Bibliography

Amundson, R. (2000). Against normal function. *Studies in History and Philosophy of Biological and Biomedical Sciences, 31*(1), 33-53.

Bobrick, B. (1995). *Knotted Tongues: Stuttering in History and the Quest for a Cure.* New York, NY: Simon & Schuster.

Brown, K., Hamner, D., Foley, S., & Woodring, J. (2009). Doing disability: Disability formations in the search for work. *Sociological Inquiry, 79*(1), 3-24.

Charlton, J.I. (1998). *Nothing About Us Without Us: Disability Oppression and Empowerment.* Berkeley, CA: University of California Press.

Crow, L. (1996). Including all of our lives: Renewing the social model of disability. In J. Morris (Ed.), *Encounters with Strangers: Feminism and Disability* (pp.135-149). London, UK: Women's Press.

DiLollo, A. & Favreau, C. (2010). Person-centered care and speech and language therapy. *Seminars in Speech and Language, 31*(2), 90-97.

Duchan, J.F. (2006). Providing a place in the new history of disabilities for communication access. *Disability Studies Quarterly, 26*(2).

Garland-Thomson, R. (2011). Misfits: A feminist materialist disability concept. *Hypatia, 26*(3), 591-609.

Jackson, E., Quesal, R., & Yaruss, J.S. (2012). What is stuttering (revisited). Paper presented at the International Stuttering Awareness Day online conference, 2012.

Kafer, A. (2013). *Feminist, Queer, Crip.* Bloomington, IA: Indiana University Press.

Loriente, C. (2009). The demedicalization of stuttering: Towards a notion of transfluency. *Journal of Stuttering Therapy, Advocacy, & Research, 3*, 131-144.

Luterman, D.M. (2016). *Counseling Persons with Communication Disorders and their Families*, 6th ed. Austin, TX: Pro Ed.

Oliver, M. (1996). *Understanding Disability: From Theory to Practice.* Basingstoke, UK: Macmillan.

Shakespeare, T. (2006). *Disability Rights and Wrongs.* New York, NY: Routledge.

Shakespeare, T. & Watson, N. (2001). The social model of disability: An outdated ideology? In *Exploring theories and expanding methodologies: Research in Social Science and Disability* (pp.9-28). Stamford, CT: Emerald Group.

Siebers, T. (2013). Disability and the theory of complex embodiment—for identity politics in a new register. In L.J. Davis (Ed.), *The Disability Studies Reader*, 4th ed. (pp.278-297). New York, NY: Routledge.

Snyder, S. L., & Mitchell, D. T. (2005). *Cultural Locations of disability*. Chicago, IL: University of Chicago Press.

St. Pierre, J. & St. Pierre, C. (2018). Governing the voice: A critical history of Speech-Language Pathology. *Foucault Studies, 24*(4), 151-184.

Van Riper, C. (1963). *Speech Correction: Principles and Methods*, 4th ed. Englewood Cliffs, NJ: Prentice-Hall.

Walker, N. (2014, September 27). Neurodiversity: Some basic terms and definitions. *Neurocosmopolitanism.*

Wilson, R.A. & St. Pierre, J. (2016). Eugenics and disability. In P. Devlieger, B. Miranda-Galarza, S.E. Brown, & M. Strickfaden (Eds), *Rethinking Disability: World Perspectives in Culture and Society* (pp.93-112). Antwerp, BE: Garant.

Wingate, M.E. (1997). *Stuttering: A Short History of a Curious Disorder*. Westport, CT: Bergin & Garvey.

Withers, A. (2012). *Disability Politics and Theory*. Winnipeg, MN: Fernwood Publishing.

Yaruss, J.S. & Quesal, R.W. (2004). Stuttering and the International Classification of Functioning, Disability, and Health: An update. *Journal of Communication Disorders, 37*(1), 35-52. doi:10.1016/S0021-9924(03)00052-2

Endnotes

[1] The charity model, for example, understands disabled people to be tragic objects of pity who need to be helped. And within the religious model, disabilities such as stuttering are taken to be a sign of divine punishment or judgement, deviation from a divine order (that will one day be made right), or sin. This chapter would also be aided by a discussion of the eugenic (Wilson & St. Pierre, 2016) and minority models (Brown, Hamner, Foley, & Woodring, 2009) of disability.

[2] The issue is a little more complex within the stuttering community because many SLPs are also people who stutter. On the one hand, stuttering SLPs are in a unique position since they have knowledge from both sides. However, I argue that stuttering SLPs actually need to work harder to counter the biases of medicalized and expert knowledge.

[3] It should be noted, however, that historically the social model largely focused on fmobility and perception disabilities at the exclusion of intellectual and developmental disabilities.

Why stutter more?

Emma Alpern

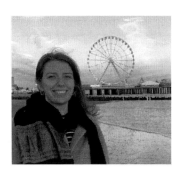

Stutterers want to not stutter, but they also want to stutter. What is this second desire? Why do our minds, our mouths, keep returning to stuttered speech? And can we find pleasure in it, since we keep wanting it, despite ourselves? Can we even start to want to stutter more?

At a bar, I lean toward the bartender to order a drink, and stutter when I say it: "Hi, how are you? Can I have a Bl-Bl-Bl-Blue Moon?" I turn to my friend and say how good it felt to stutter like that, in a one-off interaction, with that kind of a bounce. I'm surprised, because I usually don't notice the pleasures of stuttering. But there it is: my voice.

Part of it is physical: the exhilaration of stuttering, that little loss of control that resolves itself so beautifully sometimes. I am falling through the air for an instant, then catching the ground again, like Fred Astaire pretending to trip when he dances.

Part of it is about hearing my voice, and knowing others hear it too: the special stuttered fluency that belongs just to me and other stutterers. When I am fluent like non-stuttering people, I am passing, and I know it could end at any second. When I am fluent and stuttering, I am speaking as myself.

Part of it is about personal history: stuttering marks a move away from fear and shame. After years of covert stuttering, every open stutter is a hard-won victory that fills me with a feeling of pride.

And part of it is about language: When I stutter, I'm watching with curiosity the way my listener reacts – confused for an instant – and thinking about how delicate all our conversations are, how sensitive to any pause or interruption. Stuttering may give us special insight into language by breaking it open and exposing its seams.

To a stutterer, spoken words carry a dimension of meaning that's inaccessible to fluent speakers. This dimension is a site of anguish, anxiety and labour (whether that means speech therapy techniques or secondary behaviours), but it can also be a place for curiosity, insight and social connection.

Stuttering is historically understood by professionals through a medical lens, but limiting one's engagement with stuttering to these interpretations is a mistake. As a phenomenon of language, stuttering belongs as much to the arts and humanities as it does to speech pathology or even psychology. Looking at stuttering in this way can reveal deep wells of insight into the phenomenon, and into speaking and language as a whole. It may be a way to make the argument for stuttering more – an argument that seems necessary to counteract the overwhelming imperative to stutter less. How can we play with that second desire, the need to stutter? And how can we rethink its meaning to stop ourselves from understanding stuttering as brokenness?

By stuttering more, I mean something different than 'avoidance-reduction therapy' or 'effective communication' that integrates stuttering but attempts to clean it and keep its awkwardness in check. Many of us have found that embracing stuttering leads to less tension and fewer blocks, and this itself is a profound experience. I wonder if we can approach stuttering without the language of palliative care, without always associating stuttering (even 'clean' stuttering) with pain and fluency with relief.

To do so, we need to make an argument for stuttering itself. But the idea of stuttering more can appear naive or even offensive. It's easy for some of us with high natural fluency to argue for stuttering, but what about more overt stutterers who just want smoother speech so they can live their lives? I don't want to deny these experiences, but it seems important to offer an alternative. We can't let palliative arguments stop us from advocating for stuttering as a potentially enriching experience. At the same time, we should keep in mind the discomfort of stuttering and the hostility stutterers face from the fluent world. These are inextricable parts of the stuttering experience.

The project of depathologizing stuttering as a way to reduce stigma and shame becomes easier when we engage with it through a different framework: one that allows room for playfulness, for aesthetic insight, and for an analysis of stuttering's place in culture. Part of this project happens in academia and among speech-pathology professionals, but engaging with stuttering in this way is just as vital and accessible to stutterers in self-help groups, in stuttering therapy sessions, and in their daily lives.

One attempt to look at stuttering and aesthetics, by 20th-century French philosopher Gilles Deleuze, creates a window into a new way to understand the phenomenon. Stuttering's atmospheric quality, as Deleuze puts it in the essay 'He Stuttered' (1997), is like a trembling, an oscillation; the quiver, the murmur, the vibrato. These affective characteristics are linked to the speaker, but in novels, Deleuze writes, we can see how they signify more than just the speaker's speech production. Rather, "language itself stutters": it's linked to the entire atmosphere of the novel, and has significance outside of speech. "Language trembles from head to toe."

Similarly, it can be exhilarating to think of stuttering not as a speech disorder but as a phenomenon that happens within language itself, and that even improves language. Language stutters, Deleuze says, when it reaches its limit; great works of art "attain pure visions" and expose "an underside, an inverse, an inkstain or unreadable handwriting". When we stutter, we can imagine ourselves speaking at a limit, exposing the atmospheric potential of words, and bringing to the surface their strange physicality. "Everyone can talk about his memories," says Deleuze, "invent stories, state opinions in his language," but this is something else.

One example of 'something else': A stutterer at a party stands in a small group. She knows two of the people in her circle, but the three others she hasn't met yet (maybe the stutterer experiences a trembling of anticipation). After talking for a few minutes, one of the strangers reaches over to introduce herself. As they shake hands, the stutterer goes to say her name, but can't. Instead, she says something different over and over, to buy time – maybe "um" – and tries to smile as she stares into the stranger's eyes. The group realizes something is off within an instant. Their hands are still together, but they've stopped squeezing. Another three seconds pass and the stutterer glances over into the eyes of one of the people she knows, who immediately says her name for her.

When the underside of language is revealed by stuttering in this way, in the instant before saying a name, it sends an immediate shock through the listeners. In one way, it seems like speech is broken when this happens, but we may do better to understand it as simply something that happens in language. The stuttered introduction carries a unique charge that, when we step away, can almost seem exciting. And the attendant gestures – the long handshake, the glance to the friend, the nervous laughs – are also compelling, atmospheric.

While the surface of conversation may feel relatively level to most fluent speakers, to stutterers, familiar with anticipation, memories, and physical struggles, it's infused with significance. When introducing ourselves, we see the conversation from above, watch the shock our listeners receive, and navigate their responses as best we can. Stutterers, in some way, become experts at speaking.

Stuttering more can be a way to play with the drama of conversation. And when we think of stuttering as a valid thing that happens in language – 'language itself stutters' – it might become easier to experience stuttering without shame.

It might even become something we want to experience, a special dimension of conversation that we can find meaning within.

Stuttering therapy that shows us how to shape our words fluently or be 'successful communicators' will never help us access the underside of language that stuttering can reveal. Stutterers experience a uniquely embodied and passionate version of speech, but we are not usually equipped to observe it with curiosity. Rather, when we seek help, we are given ways to tamp down the strangeness of stuttering. It's essential that speech pathologists understand what language looks like to stutterers. They should do so not only so that they can help stutterers, but also because stuttering is rich with meaning in its own right, and is worth looking at - not just normalizing.

Maybe by privileging the atmospheric power of the stutter, we can resist what we've been taught to value about talking: efficiency, cleanness, and transaction. Stuttering more suggests another set of speaking values: passion, disobedience, curiosity.

References

Deleuze, G. (1997). He stuttered. In: *Essays Critical and Clinical* (pp.23-29); trans: D.W. Smith & M.A. Greco. Minneapolis, MI: University of Minnesota Press.

Scary canary: Difference, vulnerability and letting go of struggle

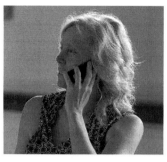

I am a happy stammerer, even on the bloomin' phone!

Katy Bailey

A canary is a delicate little bird that sings sweetly, but incessantly. In the olden days canaries were taken down coal mines because they were especially sensitive. Any toxic gases killed them first and their singing stopped, warning the miners of danger while they could still get away.

Using the social model, I will show how stammering is a canary for social toxins; whether people feel OK to stammer is an indicator of whether we are living in a safe environment. I will also suggest that stammering really is scary. Experiencing stammering as speaker or listener cuts to the chase, straight to basic existential fears, and therefore it makes sense that negative attitudes about stammering exist.

The social model of disability changed my life. The social model defines the impairment, so for stammerers our dysfluency thing, as separate from being disabled. It explains that there is a social process of disablement when a person with an impairment encounters a barrier, and that this disablement is a big part of what makes life more difficult for people who have impairments. The degree of disablement is different in different environments. Disablement is often illustrated using an example of someone with a static physical impairment like a spinal injury. If you use a wheelchair to get around, you are obviously more disabled when facing a flight of stairs rather than a lift. A stammerer has an underlying impairment, their proneness to dysfluency. How disabled you are as a stammerer depends on the barriers you encounter.

Most people who are disabled encounter negative attitudes as well as stairs and inaccessible transport. Unusually, in stammering, this is the main type of barrier we meet. There are a few physical barriers for people who stammer, for example I don't do well with computer speech recognition, but the main barriers I encounter are negative attitudes, and actions guided by these attitudes. The social model defines these negative attitudes as barriers just as real as a concrete flight of stairs, and it hurts just as much to bump into them. These negative attitudes are communicated to us in myriad subtle, and not-so-subtle, ways. But one way or another society says, "don't do that thing!". Our understandable response is to try not to do that thing.

It is interesting and useful to look at why that thing, dysfluency, freaks people out. When I got stuck talking as a child, I felt physically scared. I blocked in my larynx and my airflow would be temporarily cut off. I felt that the block might not stop, and I could die. Stammering can be scary for the stammerer. It is also challenging for the listener and for society. Dysfluent speech is noticeable and different. Lovely little children without malice often focus in on my dysfluency, saying things like, "Why can't you talk properly?" Humans are exquisitely attuned to listening for rhythm and we focus on recognizing speech from an early age, in a similar way to recognizing faces. When we encounter someone who has a very different face, what is sometimes called a facial disfigurement, we notice. We are often initially challenged and "don't know where to look". I think it is the same with stammering; dysfluent speech attracts attention because it is different. There is also a more modern analogy – in general, we don't like glitches.

A lack of control over our bodies is scary. I want my body to be reliable and do what I want when I want. If I can't control how my speech comes out maybe I can't control other actions, including keeping myself safe. Dysfluency also challenges people, and one of our seeming obsessions, in a specific way. In listening to dysfluent speech, both the listener and the person speaking are asked to wait. We only need to witness people honking at traffic lights or fidgeting and tutting in queues to realize a lot of us struggle to wait. Waiting is existentially scary, especially for modern Westerners conditioned to "want it now!". The fantasy of having control over the timing of our actions is very appealing. We are brought face-to-face with the fact that we can't speak with the reliable rhythm and timing that we want, or we find that the words don't come out at all. It is a nasty surprise; a challenge to the listener and to the speaker. Having to wait in a conversation, rather than the passing of turns and time going the way you expect, is disconcerting.

At various times in my life, I have feared silence. The worst silence was the screaming, ear-piercing silence of my own blocks. I was worried that someone would fill my turn in the conversation and maybe even in life. I was scared that I, and we, might be stuck forever. A lack of control in relationship with time reminds us that we are all powerless to prevent the ticking of the clock;

we will age and die, and likely not at a moment of our choosing. Dysfluency shouts out that we are imperfect and vulnerable. We are delicate human bodies, vulnerable like a small bird who will fade and perish. In general, people don't want to be reminded of their mortality, especially not unexpectedly in the street or on the phone.

Finding a difference initially surprising, and even deeply challenging, is understandable. But what happens next? As the exposure is challenging it is understandable that people may want to avoid and not engage with it. We don't want to see or know the scary truth about bodies. This can lead to a physical difference being labelled by the individual or by society as 'bad', so a negative attitude to facial or speech difference develops. These attitudes can shape how people behave and communicate with the person who is defined as different and 'bad'. Some people with facial differences are subject to abuse, including suggestions that they shouldn't show their faces. People whose speech sounds different are also subject to actions driven by the negative attitudes held by others.

Negative attitudes to stammering exist; this is just an unpleasant fact. It is natural that we as people who stammer absorb and come to share these dominant attitudes and act accordingly. This is called internalized oppression, or self-stigma. Many of us can't remember a time before we knew we should try not to do that thing. In many families, including my own, the stammering thing was not named or spoken about openly, but it was certainly communicated; I knew it upset my parents and, in my childhood brain, that meant it was bad.

And we all know what happens next, that child will push, take a run up, take another breath, or clash their teeth, use 'sort of, sort of, sort of' fillers, or avoid the word or speaking altogether. In other words, they struggle. This struggle is on top of the underlying dysfluency. It is something we do as a response to the negative attitudes we perceive, and as such it is the process of disablement in action.

I am particularly interested in discussing the noises we make when we struggle, but there is a range of responses from noisy struggle to silent avoidance. I include avoidance behaviours in my definition of struggle. They are part of the same process. For me, struggle is everything we do, often very inventive and sometimes extreme, to try not to stammer, essentially to avoid experiencing or showing the moment of dysfluency. I used to push, hard! For example, repeating an already uttered sound like a machine gun in order to propel myself past a sound I feared I would stammer on. I also used to dislocate my jaw with an audible click and throw my head back, sometimes into walls.

Let's get back to the social model. Our underlying impairment, our basic level of dysfluency, is cloaked, enveloped and sometimes completely obscured by the disabling process itself. In response to the attitudinal barriers we encounter, our efforts 'not to do that thing' are enacted in struggle behaviour. But this struggle sounds like, and is often defined by others as, more of our underlying impairment. By misattributing our greater struggle to a worsening in our dysfluency, they fail to appreciate the role of greater hostility in the environment. The underlying dysfluency (our impairment) and our struggle (the disablement process) are both called stammering; they are conflated.

Many people who stammer are perplexed by how variable their stammering is; for some this can be the most confusing and painful aspect. The fact that stammering is variable, and is a behaviour (something we do), makes it very easy to think that stammering is all about us as an individual, all our own personal problem. I remember berating myself that my stammer was different in different environments – "Why can't I just talk like I do on my own in my bedroom?" This is a double bind, a tortuous catch-22. This conflation of dysfluency (our impairment) and struggle (the disablement process) in stammering means it is really difficult for people who stammer to unpick what is going on, to recognize the mechanism through which we are disabled by our interactions with attitudinal barriers.

Let's look more at these negative attitudes. We grow up with them, they are around us in the classroom, playground, and media. I was taunted at school for stammering. I was scared of the telephone ringing and scared to say my name. I knew stammering was a bad thing and I hoped and wished it would go away.

As an undergraduate student, I went to Jamaica for three months to study. Whilst there, I pretty much stopped stammering; it certainly stopped being a problem. As soon as I arrived I started to receive overtly positive reactions to my dysfluency: "Oh, you stammer like my cousin!", or "You are the first white person I have met who stammers!" accompanied by smiling faces and friendly interest. Dysfluency became a positive attribute. There seemed to be quite a lot of stammering in Jamaica and it was talked about freely. I stopped being worried how people would respond to my stammering; I stopped trying not to stammer.

When I returned to England my stammering gradually returned. A notable response brought me back down to earth. I was talking about stammering feeling less of an issue and a university lecturer retorted, "That's all very well, but you'll have to be fluent in your finals!"

Unfortunately, negative attitudes to stammering are also present when we, or our parents, eventually ask for some help from the health visitor, family doctor, or at school. Negative attitudes to dysfluency also exist in the speech therapy profession. I remember being at a conference and another speaker, a speech therapist, returned to her seat after her presentation and anxiously asked her colleague, "Was I really dysfluent?" Heaven forbid!

It has been fashionable in speech therapy for people who stammer to be told that "listeners don't mind stammering", often as an attempt to make them feel more relaxed. Whilst it is true that some people don't mind stammering, and it is true that most people could learn to not mind stammering, it is a lie to say that negative attitudes to stammering do not exist or are not communicated; it negates the lived experience of people who stammer to pretend this is so. Having my lived experience negated does not make me feel more relaxed. It is true that, when asked, lots of people will say they don't mind stammering… but many people would also deny their racism or homophobia.

Negative attitudes exist and are communicated, and there is also the issue of perception. Being sensitive to damaging stimuli is natural. It is true that many people who stammer become very sensitive to negative attitudes to stammering, in the same way that gazelles become sensitive, even hypersensitive, to lions. Sensitized perception is part of the disabling process; it is an internalized expectation of a negative reaction. This is based on past negative experience, and the ongoing relationship between this and our internalized oppression means we can even come to think we deserve a negative reaction and we may even provide a negative reaction for ourselves if it is not forthcoming from others. These are all elements of disablement in action. I have met some people who do not seem very attuned to the responses of others, people who are very dysfluent and yet show no signs of struggle or avoidance. They appear not in the slightest bit bothered by the reaction of others, and their speaking is less of a problem to them; consequently, they are less disabled.

Part of reducing the disablement process in action, the struggle and avoidance, is to work directly on our sensitized perceptions of negative attitudes, and indeed to work directly on our internalized oppression. There are good ways to achieve this; there is a lot to learn from happy stammerers. Crucially though, this approach of focusing on the stammerer only works when linked with work on reducing actual negative attitudes outside the stammerer.

In the summer of 2014, I had reached a point of truly accepting myself and that it was OK to stammer. I had been lucky enough to get some brilliant help at the City Lit in London to let go of my struggle. I wanted to share my thoughts and I was happy to be invited to work together with speech therapist

Sam Simpson and another person who stammers, St John Harris. We wrote a presentation and went to the Oxford Dysfluency Conference, the big international professional conference for speech therapists and researchers. That day rocked me to the core. I have only recently analyzed what happened; at the time, I did the metaphorical version of running away as fast as I could. I was on the brink of writing some more good stuff with that team and I did a complete 180; I turned away from all things stammery. Looking back, my newfound acceptance of myself was shaken. I had willingly gone into an environment that communicated loudly to me that I was a bad thing. Researchers were proudly presenting their work, on successes during the 'curable phase', subjecting toddlers to MRI scans to map the brain pathology in stammering, unethical behavioural work with children, and progress towards finding the gene. I was witnessing a wonderful excitement that pervaded the whole conference about finding the gene! Finding the gene may be interesting scientifically, but it also paves the way for prenatal testing and deciding which foetuses get born, so there don't need to be people like me anymore. That way lies eugenics and worse. I could hear the Scary Canary's voice weakening. I was a walking, talking, stammering personification of failure for many people at that conference. I hadn't been aborted, I hadn't been cured during the golden window and I hadn't engaged properly with effective fluency shaping regimes... and what's more I had the cheek to say I was happy about it! Being in that environment made me question again whether it was OK to stammer. It didn't feel very OK to stammer and that feeling was all too familiar from my earlier life. So, I ran away.

In November 2016, I came back to talking and writing about stammering. I came back because I want to stand up and say, "I am OK and I won't be oppressed". I won't have myself defined as someone else's failed project. I am back because I know the difference between oppressive and liberating speech therapy and I want us to be open about what is right and wrong.

So, truth time. Some therapies are oppressive. For me, communicating to people who stammer that they should, or even could, be fluent is oppressive. It is understandable that helping people who say they really want to be fluent try to be fluent seems like an uncomplicated endeavour. Except remember how internalized oppression works... in the early 20th century, some black people really didn't want to be black and until recently some gay people really didn't want to be gay. I am happy to say that treatments for these perceived 'problems' are no longer available on the National Health Service, at least not in the UK. It can be seen as oppressive that a profession (at least historically) based on fixing us exists at all. I admit I look forward to the day when Fluency Specialist does not exist as a job. However, I want to hold out a hand of friendship and partnership in speech therapy work because many people who stammer in Britain continue to suffer; some people who stammer are disabled to a terrible degree and we can certainly do with some helpful help. We need to be less disabled by society. This means reducing barriers, but it also means naming struggle as part of the disabling process. It means no longer conflating underlying dysfluency with struggle; not throwing the innocent baby of dysfluency out with the dirty bathwater of struggle.

Unhelpful help is the most insidious kind of oppression. It is oppressive to try to eradicate impairment, especially when the impairment is or can be painless. It is the worst kind of disablism to try to eradicate painless impairment just so 'normal' people don't have to hear it. My underlying stammer, my basic dysfluency with the struggle largely offloaded, is not painful. People who stammer will have different levels of underlying dysfluency, but even if we discover that our underlying dysfluency is frequent and regular, it does not have to be painful in the way that struggle to not stammer is painful.

Although well meant, it is oppressive to collude with someone's internalized oppression by not exploring what is behind their understandable first wish "just to be fluent", or even by supporting an option of aiming to eradicate dysfluency. Good speech therapists can use all their skills and knowledge with so much more power once we jettison the bigotry against dysfluency. There are many skills used in fluency work that will be more effective when used to work only on reducing struggle, once the fear of underlying impairment is reduced or removed.

Acknowledging that negative attitudes exist gives speech therapy work context and gives people who stammer space to think about what it really is that feels difficult about stammering. A person has an underlying dysfluency and, in an environment that includes negative attitudes about dysfluency, a disablement process occurs where they are motivated to struggle or avoid. Identifying that this process exists can be liberating. My struggling is amenable to change supported by liberating speech therapy. Helping people discover and engage with their dysfluency, beneath the struggling, is rewarding work. This type of therapy is enjoyed by the best stammering therapists. However, it all goes to waste if the same skills are used oppressively, even with the best intentions, against the underlying, natural dysfluency or difference.

Once the barrage of noisy struggle is eased, the small quiet voice of the Scary Canary must not be snuffed out too. Therapists are sabotaging themselves and their clients by succumbing to the oppressive ideal of fluency. If you are pushed to pursue fluency at all costs you lose your real voice and spontaneity; something valuable, indeed priceless. You will never lose your fear of stammering if your listeners, including your therapist and yourself, view dysfluency as failure. Fluency, as an idealized complete absence of dysfluency, is a myth in the live version of life, like perfect anything. What feels lovely is speaking spontaneously and freely, without being judged as bad. This is available for all people who stammer once the disablement process stops.

Reducing disablement is mostly about raising awareness, changing attitudes and preventing the enactment of discrimination fuelled by these attitudes. We need to get people who don't stammer to change their behaviours and attitudes. As discussed, these negative attitudes are explainable on the individual and social level, and I suggest they are fuelled by powerful existential fears. This means they will probably not melt away conveniently; this is big stuff.

With all discussions of disability using the social model, we are thinking about how the environment can be changed to reduce barriers. For children and adults, the main thing that helps or hinders is listener response. We can raise awareness that dysfluency exists and raise awareness that, although it might be natural to be surprised and discombobulated when you hear dysfluency, it is not OK to laugh, copy, make fun of or discriminate against the person, or edit out dysfluency. Helpful things include hearing more dysfluent voices in common speaking roles, as teachers, religious leaders and in customer services, and in the media; challenging the practice of editing the dysfluency out of recorded speech (did you even know this happens routinely?). This will help because people who stammer, including children, will hear that they are 'not the only one' and that most people are dysfluent sometimes. Also, for those who don't stammer, it gives the opportunity to experience their natural reactions to hearing dysfluent speech. They can work through it and realize that, to steal from a fabulous advertising campaign, "some people stammer, get over it!". I never want to be the first stammerer anyone hears. I want everyone to have engaged with an important aspect of civilized socialization, meeting all their peers in inclusive education and seeing and hearing people with a range of different attributes, including impairments, in the media.

Acknowledging that negative attitudes to dysfluency exist allows the person who stammers to understand why they are so primed to struggle against dysfluency. Naming this struggle as part of the disablement process gives us the power to change it. I don't want to be just another voice asking people who stammer to change their behaviour, God knows we've had enough of that! As I've said, I am mostly asking people who don't stammer to change their behaviour and ideally their attitudes. However, I am inviting people who stammer to look at their struggle, with the support of a liberating speech therapist if that helps. In the same way that we encourage young people wondering about their sexuality or being bullied for the colour of their skin not to hide away in their bedrooms and wish themselves different, let's encourage our people to accept and show their stammers, their real stammers with the layers of struggle, the disablement process, gently loosened away. I believe that everyone who stammers can find their basic level of dysfluency underneath all the struggle; dysfluent speech that is the least physically distressing.

Because of the complex nature of struggle, there is still a place for liberating therapy to help people who stammer become less disabled; that is to identify, remove, reduce, and negotiate the barriers they encounter in life. This is best done in groups where people who stammer can recognize their shared experience and be strengthened by this recognition. In my case, when I named what I was doing as struggle the change followed quite naturally. I realized my struggling was incongruent with my core belief that it's OK to stammer. The next step was realizing I wanted to struggle less, that it's OK not to struggle. There is a habitual aspect to struggle; I had been doing it for a long time. I had also become practised at turning off my self-awareness in the moment of struggling. I was helped at the City Lit to become more aware, to become mindful during my struggling and let my dysfluency show. It is not an easy task, though; showing our underlying stammering can feel scary, especially initially. Although futile, we may have been holding onto our struggle to avoid accepting that our stammering was real or accepting the vulnerability of having to wait for our speech, maybe being scared to expose our Scary Canary to the world. Maybe thinking that one day we might win; I know I held on tight to the fight. As you can't 'overcome' struggle, I had to agree a truce and let go. Once I had experienced dysfluent speech without struggle it became less scary. I found I could demand that my dysfluency, my natural speech, my Scary Canary, was accepted. The good news is that getting together and campaigning with other people who stammer is a powerful fuel for these positive but difficult changes.

The most important thing is changing behaviour in the general public and in people with the power to discriminate. Hopefully, attitude change will follow this. We can all do this, especially influential people such as parents, teachers and speech therapists. We can change attitudes by proudly being ourselves. It is essential, I believe, to accept that we do have an underlying impairment, our dysfluency-prone speech. That's it. It's not too bad. It's an

OK thing to accept and something that will never stop us doing anything we want, except elite fluency sports. Bloody elite fluency sports! The realm of competitive sport often concerns elite versions of those physical abilities which are affected by impairment. Moving, strength, running, dexterity, thinking and speaking clearly, doing things perfectly without shaking or wobbling and most of all doing things for a long time or fast... we return to the allure of mastering rhythm and time. The thing I can't do is talk as fast as a fast, fluent speaker. Get your stopwatch out and I will not win. I am not elite at speaking.

In the stammering world, there is beginning to be talk of the advantages of stammering and, whilst I now see my dysfluency, my reclaimed stammering, as a positive in my life, I think it is a mistake to mimic the very attitudes that disable so many people. We don't need to turn stammering into something that makes us 'better than other people' in order to be proud. We don't need to be 'superheroes overcoming adversity'. We just need to be allowed to be ourselves with our stammery speech. It is much more powerful to be asserting that it is OK to be different and even measurably worse at things. The pride that changes society is saying it is OK, it is fabulous, simply to be a type of real person. That I, and you, have equal value just for being people. This is when society starts getting seriously good.

Let's talk about self-acceptance. Acceptance is great but let's not jump to it too quickly. In another horrible twist, the fashion for self-acceptance can become another tool of oppression. Do you remember the problem with the conflation of the underlying dysfluency and the disablement process of struggle, that they are often both called stammering? If we decide, or are encouraged, to 'just accept our stammering' we can tie ourselves up in knots thinking we should be able to accept a stammer that we find, and that really is, unacceptable. We can even beat ourselves up all over again for not 'accepting it properly enough'. A stammer that is so full of struggle as to be causing physical pain, making us breathless to the point of light-headedness or damaging our teeth is not acceptable; it's not OK to hurt ourselves, it is not OK to accept oppression. Being made to feel bad for not accepting oppression? That really is weird, and wrong!

So, when you reduce the disablement process what does this struggle-free dysfluency feel like? Underlying levels of dysfluency vary. In the past, my full-of-struggle stammering was severe at times despite realizing later that my underlying level of dysfluency is low. I used to worry about my stammering many times a day, desperately hoping it would stop, or that I could find more energy for the fight. Nowadays, weeks can go by without a worry about my speech. I will stammer anywhere! I stammer in groups at work, I just reach out and stammer on the telephone and even at my wedding, they couldn't get the microphone off me. I am a happy stammerer. I have let go of my inflated ideals of fluency, let go of my gold medal hopes in those elite fluency sports and accepted my different sounding speech; that which I previously considered bad.

Underlying dysfluency remains out of our control and is therefore still scary. However, we can learn to do scary things and be brave; brave enough to speak spontaneously and stammer, voluntarily if necessary. Stammering on purpose is a particularly powerful personal and political action. When I was a teenager, speaking fluently using a fluency technique used to sound good to others but felt terrifying for me, like walking along a high wire above an applauding audience. I felt like I had so far to fall, back to the shameful failure of stammering. I believe this is an unavoidable problem with fluency techniques. If you are constantly winning against your stammering there is always the risk that one day you may lose again. Stammering on purpose, voluntary stammering, along with letting our underlying dysfluency show, transports that tightrope right down to the ground. There is nowhere to fall because I am doing and showing what I used to be so scared of. I can walk freely, fall around a bit, and the audience can clap or not if they feel like it. My talking no longer feels like such high-wire performance and there is no fear of failing at talking.

I think dysfluency is beautiful. A flower is beautiful because it holds within it the inevitable promise of decay and death, not despite this. Our lives are precious because we will inevitably fade and die. It is tempting to fool ourselves that we are invulnerable or immortal, and goodness knows there are enough companies trying to sell us the promise of beating ageing. When I pay attention to my dysfluent speech I am brought face-to-face with my frail humanity, as are my listeners. The Scary Canary has an important song to sing. This exposure to existential truths is uncomfortable initially but is also that which can save us from the spiralling toxic by-products of a futile race against basic existential facts, including mortality. We could exhaust our energies in a difficult and dirty world by chasing the impossible dream of invulnerability, whether through numbing consumerism or through the seemingly rising drive to park scary 'badness' in those who are deemed different and other. We are better when we remember we are all humans together, we all eat, digest, shit, grow old and die... and we all breathe the same air.

In 2016, I went somewhere that felt very different to Oxford; I went to the Manchester British Stammering Association conference. I was no longer among only a few voices talking about the social model and pride and it felt great. There were choruses of Scary Canaries singing proudly, showing our stammering and demanding to be listened to. I came home knowing the future of stammering in this country is safe in the hands of the next generation and that I can play my part too.

Pride is reclaiming what society has historically defined as bad, and part of pride is demanding to be the ones who theorize and produce knowledge about our dysfluency. In other words, 'nothing about us without us'. It is time for us to work together: stammerers, charities, the disabled people's movement, educators, and speech therapist allies. In collaboration, we can design a different model for reducing the disablement experienced by people who stammer. It is all about communicating that it is OK to stammer, and it is OK to let go of struggle. As well as raising awareness of stammering and encouraging behavioural change in listeners and organizations, this needs to include the removal of oppressive therapy and increase of support for people who stammer to let go of struggle. Part of the plan would be making high-quality, evidence-based, and effective liberating speech therapy available around the country. I would like to invite all SLTs to become SLTs all over again: Struggle and Liberation Therapists. This liberating therapy needs to be inextricably linked to people who stammer getting together for peer support, recognizing pride, and doing the thinking and campaigning that will fuel our liberation. Speech therapists can enable and encourage peer support, but they can't be part of it, unless they are lucky enough to be stammerers too!

Back to the canary. What would happen if there were no Scary Canaries, if we never heard people speaking dysfluently? We might be more able to fool ourselves that our bodies were reliable, that there was no risk in life, and we were invulnerable. We wouldn't know how toxic our society was becoming until it was too late and eventually even the fittest suffocated. Let's keep the stammering canary singing loudly and proudly as this shows us we're living somewhere where it's OK to be different; where the air is clean enough to breathe and speak, in our own way.

Time-Bound

Nisar Bostan

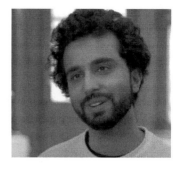

Featuring on 'The Undateables' was my claim to fame.

My thoughts spiral in flitter array,
confused by the anarchy caused by my enunciation.

My words become an incoherent dollop,
an exodus of stillborn syllables and words,
obsolete when most pined,
the infatuation of fluency a fleeting one.

I tentatively scour the room I am sat in,
tacitly probing the sea of familiar faces,
my aural senses rekindled by the inevitable sound of half-suppressed
snickering.

Eerie silence ensues, encapsulating my audience...

The barter of sheepish stares offers little in the way of penance,
the impotent feeling of inferiority relishing in its sovereignty,
the wrath of my inner-self and fortitude dearly interrogated.

Their patience wanes...

I am intermittently disrupted mid-sentence,
the room abuzz with secular rapport once again,
my facial contortions and rasping breath left fledgling in rhetoric disarray.

I am relegated into the abyss.

My name is Nisar Bostan.

I have a stammer.

My cursive writing vouches for the conversations that are never had,
an unsatiating desire to substitute the words I stutter on with curt synonyms,
my vocabulary a masquerade to avoid hasty generalisations.

I am not a stammerer, yet I stammer.

I am not disabled, yet others disable me.

I am not a label, yet others label me.

I am what I am; I am not what I am.

Objectivity reigns above subjectivity,
apathy compromises empathy,
unambiguity reprises ambiguity.

Stammering is suppressing, but yet it is... liberating.

Obscuring my stammer is easy, but yet it is... hard.

Conforming to mainstream society is conventional, but yet it is... unconventional.

Dichotomies that I have become all too used to.

I yearn for a truce between my mind and heart.

I find myself walking on eggshells,
caught in-between two stools,

grey matter meshed with "should it even matter?"

After all are we not all expatriates waiting to be repatriated,
biding time until it is finally our time?

From the outside-in,

I may seem to be going through the motions,
going through life,
but look a little closer,
and with each conversation shared,

I am growing through life.

Me and you are similar,
bogged down by the same predicament,
vying to personify and dignify our thoughts in a society geared towards
insincere glib and fibs.

Is that even fair for those whose dysfluency acts as a red-herring?!

My spiel is no self-proclaimed "Art",
but a tactic to avoid succumbing to semantics,
an affirmation unto myself
not in need of anyone's validation.

My stammer offers a modicum of hope,
an epitome of sincerity, integrity and compassion,

I am unique and idiosyncratic in my own queer nature.

We all are.

I may be a little unorthodox,

I may be a little disillusioned,
incessantly convincing myself that my imperfections are my perfections.

I may take longer to muster words than others.

But most importantly...

I do have needs.

I do have emotions.

I do feel vulnerable.

And I do feel insecure.

Writing may be my medium of catharsis,

...

But I DO have a voice.

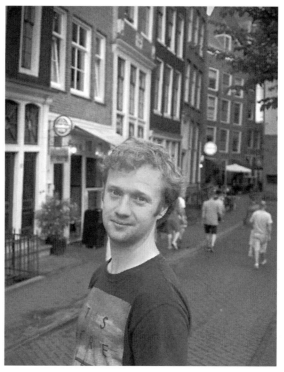

A friend who stammers took this photo of me in Amsterdam after a stammering youth meeting in Holland in 2014; it is my go to photo to this day.

People with stigma: A reflection on stigma against stammering in society and the stammerer

Patrick Campbell

Life as a person who stammers is difficult. The stammered voice is out of place in our fast-paced, fluency-oriented society, and people who stammer feel the consequences. There are subtle moments of exclusion, such as a verbal wrestling match with a voice automated telephone system, to outright discrimination, such as the bullying of a child who stammers at school. There is shame and struggle.

We have a tendency to place the blame for these negative feelings and experiences on stammering itself. I used to. It is easy to think that if people who stammer could just be fluent, like the rest of society, then these moments of exclusion and discrimination would not happen. Yet this superficial and reductive line of thinking stops us from asking deeper and more profound questions about the fairness and inclusivity of our society towards the natural diversity of the human species. What if the problem lies not with the person who stammers' way of speaking but rather society's reaction to it?

I was a slow convert to this social model way of thinking, but I have found power in repositioning personal responsibility for my difficulties with stammering onto society. I want to share that with you. I want to explore how I feel society is to blame for the difficulties people who stammer have through life: how stigma against stammering is widespread, how the world is subtly set up to disadvantage people who stammer and how, consequently, people who stammer can come to live their life with a pervasively negative, but unwarranted, view of their own speech. I believe people who stammer are better understood as people with stigma rather than people with a speech problem.

Chris and Sam, my fellow editors, thought this chapter was more loose than the other I worked on. I agree. It is an incomplete mish-mash of formal research, lived experience and personal theories. I would be interested to hear what you think as you go, in particular the moments and images of stigma that come into your own head: because stigma occurs by a thousand cuts and my chapter only manages to find a few incisions. There are a lot more. It will need our collective considered reflection to perceive them, for only then can they be challenged.

> "How do we recognise the shackles that tradition has placed on us? For if we can recognise them, we are able to break them." – Franz Boas

What is the problem with stammering?

I often think of my first year of medical training. I spent most of my time that year trying to avoid stammering. I used a catalogue of tricks that are well-known to people who stammer, from word swapping to avoiding roles that involved speaking at length. I used these tricks to appear to be the fluent, articulate communicator I thought I needed to be to become a doctor. Ironically, they made me a worse communicator: I did not say what I wanted to and I often spoke in convoluted and confusing sentences.

I wish I had thought this through. What part of stammering makes a person who stammers incapable of being a doctor? Sure, if you stammer in a consultation it might take a bit longer, but as long as the patient keeps listening and the environment is supportive there is no change in the person's ability as a doctor. The same diagnosis is made and the same treatment is given by a doctor who stammers[1].

We have such a focus on stammering as a problem or defect in society that we never consider what this supposed problem is at heart. The 'problem' appears to me to be a tendency to make people wait longer when communicating and concentrate a bit more[2]. It is not life or death.

> "The stutter itself is only a negative bodily development if making people occasionally wait an extra 2 to 10 minutes is a pathological emergency" – Zaharia Richter.

Stammering as a problem (if it even is a problem) is much more easily remedied by patience and supportive changes to the environment than the individual who stammers spending months or years of their life attempting to fix their speech to the fluent normal. This can be contemplated under the social or political model but, to me, it is also after some thought, logical.

Stigma against stammering in society

Sadly, the world does not agree with my logical deduction. Humans are a tribal species and, as history reminds us at every turn, a trait that sets an individual apart from the rest of a tribe has the potential to be the subject of prejudice and discrimination. Stammering is one of these traits; society places a value on fluency and denigrates anyone who does not live up to this norm.

The pervasive negative view of stammering and people who stammer in society has been researched at length, in particular by Kenneth St. Louis and Michael Boyle. One study that strikes me from 1997, in which a group of nurses were given a questionnaire to rate a made-up doctor. In half the cases the doctor was a fluent doctor and in the other half a doctor who stammers – no other changes were made to the questionnaire. The doctor who stammers was rated as being:

> "... more afraid, tense, nervous, and aggravating in addition to being less mature, intelligent, secure, competent, confident, educated, and reputable than a physician who does not stutter." - Silverman and Bongey (1997)

Quite a list and this is just one study... Many studies have been conducted on different populations and individuals from all walks of life and they have all converged on the opinion that the public holds attitudes about people who stammer that are biased, stigmatizing and discriminatory. Most often, society sees people who stammer as weak, less confident and less able. Maybe I was right to try to pass as fluent in medical school?

> "It is likely that if you have never been regarded as a stutterer, you can come nowhere near appreciating the uncanny, crushing power of the social disapproval of whatever is regarded as stuttering. It is probably one of the most frightening, perplexing, and demoralizing influences to be found in our culture." - Wendell Johnson

A world designed for fluency

This pervasive stigma towards stammering in turn shapes the day-to-day environment which we inhabit. The world has been designed with only the fluent in mind and it penalizes people who are not able to meet this norm. The way in which each individual who stammers is affected by this set-up is unique[3]; however, I am going to pick out common obstacles for people who stammer in this 'world designed for fluency' that stand out to me. Some are clear-cut and easy to understand, while others are more intangible. There are many more out there, but I hope these will get your own thoughts flowing.

Voice-automated systems

Voice interfaces, like Siri and Amazon Echo, are becoming more common in society. They aim to make life easier for people, making us more connected and informed. For people who stammer, however, they can do anything but this. I recently worked in a hospital that used voice recognition software to make phone calls (for example, you would have to say into the phone "Call Cardiology Doctor"). I had to pass as fluent to make the call or else go through a time-consuming process of calling a person on the switchboard to then forward the call. A verbal wrestling match with the telephone was not uncommon. The hospital voice automated phone system was designed with fluent individuals in mind; it had little accessibility to those who stammer. Communication systems are being built for the vast majority of people at the centre point of a bell curve of fluent speech. This leaves people who stammer on the edges of this new technological society.

'Fluent communication skills required'

The job adverts are clear: excellent, fluent communication skills are required to succeed in the business place. I would go further and say fluent communication skills are required to succeed in everyday life. Many of our daily interactions are designed to be quick and efficient without interruption. Think of interactions at supermarkets, train station kiosks and banks: these are assumed to happen in fast, fluent tongue. Stammering has the habit of disrupting these activities. This leads to servers becoming impatient and annoyed and people who stammer feeling rushed and under pressure, as the normal interactional patterns and expectations of our society are interrupted.

A fair society designed for people who stammer would make space for daily interactions to be interrupted by dysfluent speech. For example, consumer-facing staff would be trained in how to interact with people who stammer and job interviewers would naturally make space for stammered speech – without the necessity of a long-debated request for extra time. Stammered speech would be included in society as an equal mode of communication.

Hidden disability

The disabling design faults of our society are harder to perceive for a hidden and variable disability like stammering than they are for physical disabilities. This has meant that, whilst activists with physical disabilities have had significant and prominent successes in changing society's design flaws to meet their differences, stammering has by and large been left off the diversity and inclusion agenda. Stammering is not perceived as a significant disability in the public eye so supportive allowances are not proactively made for it. This is perhaps in part due to society's stigma towards it, but also the tendency and ability of people who stammer to be able to pass as normal/near-normal speakers for long enough periods to seemingly surmount any systemic barriers worthy of a formal challenge. Society does not feel the need to provide a ramp for people who stammer; rather, it still expects us to limp up the stairs using our moments of fluency to act like a normal speaker.

When I was at medical school I applied for support with stammering at the disability office. What I remember most about the process was not proving that I stammered but proving that stammering was a disability. I was faced with a long form asking what disability I had, detailing many forms of disability, such as physical, hearing, reading, but none for stammering/communication. I ended up in a box entitled 'Other disability – please explain in text below' and trying to justify my application.

> "When stuttering is brought to the fore, it is often not interpreted as a "severe" disability, that is, society does not discriminate against stuttering as a whole (nor recognize it through funding and support) to the same degree that it does many other forms of physical and mental disabilities. While much of this likely has to do with the stutterer's wily ability to go incognito, often passing within society, it still causes one to wonder how much discrimination is required to be classified as disabled. In this sense, I am hesitant to place stuttering categorically alongside more visible disabilities. Yet, in the same breath, stuttering comes under distinct social pressures and punishments absent from the experience of clearly defined and visible disabilities." - Joshua St. Pierre

Role models

The role models we have for people who stammer reflect society's stereotyped and negative views of stammering. As a child, I remember being told by speech and language therapists about successful people who stammer: "People who stammer can succeed in life and become celebrities, Patrick. There is Samuel L. Jackson, Rowan Atkinson, and Bruce Willis". Now, I do like 'Pulp Fiction', adore 'Mr Bean', and I truly believe 'Die Hard' is the best Christmas film of all time, but not one of these individuals was a helpful role model for young me. Stammering for these celebrities is their broken wing start to life from which they have recovered; it is not a core part of their identity. The people we hold up to inspire children who stammer, ironically, further unhelpful tropes and attitudes towards stammering.

We need to be careful because even people who stammer and their allies can become complicit in continuing this motif. Our society is easily inspired by a story of a person 'overcoming' their speech problem. If we play into this archetype we can win superficial praise and exposure from society, but it leaves us as poorer role models to the next generation of children who stammer.

Another side-issue to this is the portrayal of characters who stammer in movies and plays. It is interesting to reflect on the furore over the 'whitewashing' of films. Society is beginning to question the rights of a white actor to play a historically non-white character and in doing so appropriate their culture without their consent. This concept has spread to physical disability with questions beginning to be asked when disabled characters are played by able-bodied actors, 'cripping-up'. Yet, such issues have rarely been mentioned in relation to stammering. Fluent actors have been freely allowed to appropriate our stammering behaviours and culture and then interpret them with artistic license to gain the most drama or laughs on the biggest stages society has to offer.

The language of the majority

The language we commonly hear, read, and speak is from a society that is predominantly fluent and holds stigmatized negative views of people who stammer. It is unsurprising, therefore, to find that the words used to describe stammering are often negative (e.g., afflicted, struggle). Some words may initially sound positive (e.g., overcome) but have subtle oppressive connotations. This may appear to be simply semantics, but this language has a large effect on society and people who stammer; it is the fabric of societal stigma against stammering.

The ubiquitous 'overcome' remains my personal nemesis. Particularly favoured by fluent newspaper writers, it holds people who stammer up as inspiration porn to the masses for defeating our 'great weakness'.

> "I view phrases such as "overcoming your stammer" or "conquering your disfluency" with suspicion – such language comes from the same ignorant and/or cruel mindset that says we lack will-power. The military metaphor turns stammerers into perpetual losers in a battle which we're too crap ever to win." – David Mitchell

This same negative language comes to be spoken by, and perhaps more importantly internalized, by people who stammer. Indeed, we think, process and consider with the language at our disposal. If a person's vocabulary around stammering is entirely negative, they will internally interpret their life experiences as a speaker in a stigmatized light. Nietzsche saw language as our prison-house, as we are unable to think beyond the boundaries of the words we know. With our current vocabulary on stammering, people who stammer remain trapped in a lexical prison.

The internalization of stigma

People who stammer talk a lot about prisons and chains, and often a feeling of 'holding back'. My mind drifts to a poem by Rosalind Harvey (2003).

> 'How can I begin to tell you this tale,
>
> of a life-serving prisoner in this puzzling jail?
>
> A jail with no shackles, no whips and no chains -
>
> But a jailer most wicked who never refrains
>
> From a continual strapping of words to the soul -
>
> A legacy of suffering is his only goal.
>
> His testing and teasing, his taunts and his lies,
>
> and unkind regard for the need of replies,
>
> I question him curtly, "when will I be free?"
>
> The jailer turns slowly - the jailer is me.'

> Rosalind Harvey

I think all this talk of prisons, chains, jailers and holding back is really an attempt to convey the power that internalized stigma, also known as 'self-stigma', can have over our lives. You see, in this melting pot of prejudice and discrimination towards stammering, people who stammer can come to absorb negative beliefs about their speech and apply them to themselves.

Self-stigma is thought about in three stages of de-valuing ourselves: awareness, agreement, and application of stereotypes. The individual first becomes aware of a stereotype about their stigmatized condition (I realized that society believed stammering showed weakness in a doctor). Over time they come to agree with that stereotype (I came to believe stammering was a sign of weakness in a doctor), and, finally, they come to apply it to themselves (I came to think I would be unable to be a doctor as a person who stammers).

The consequences of self-stigma are borne out in behaviour, and in particular for stammering 'avoidance behaviours'. As people who stammer, we can come to oppress our own stammered voice: holding it back and keeping it in chains. We avoid words that will cause us to stammer, we do not take on roles that require a lot of speaking and, ultimately, we hold back a bit of ourselves that we feel the world does not want to see.

I always feel Rosalind's poem. For me, the poem is so painful because the person is in the depths of self-hatred for what they perceive as their own actions in life. I know this feeling: a feeling of self-blame for avoiding and holding back in life. After all, I made the choice to swap words. I made the choice to avoid speaking. It is my fault that I did not always live openly as a person who stammers. On reflection, this is a misattribution of blame, a bit like victim-blaming in sexual assault cases. Having a powerful internal locus of control is commendable, but such 'avoidance behaviours' are the end result of a societal process of stigmatization of stammering – they are neither the personal fault nor autonomous decision of the person who stammers. This poem is so painful because the person is oblivious to their actual 'jailer', the stigma and shame they have internalized from the hostile environment which surrounds them.

The cure for stigma: Pride

I worry we are trapped in a vicious circle of stigma. That the processes of stigma and self-stigma lead people who stammer to turn into the very stereotypes society has preconceived of them. This then reinforces those stereotypes to society, to repeat again with the next generation.

Fortunately, people who stammer and their allies are stronger than this hypothesized vicious circle. I have met people who stammer who are energized by this widespread prejudice rather than oppressed by it. Life may be difficult for people who stammer, but it can be difficult on our own terms. We challenge societal prejudices and we have begun to build a narrative of positivity and empowerment around stammering.

These empowered, angry, energized voices are the ones you will find in the rest of this book.

"To be yourself in a world that is constantly trying to make you something else is the greatest accomplishment." - Ralph Waldo Emerson

Recommended further reading and references

Boyle, M. (2015). The importance of challenging the public stigma of stuttering. Paper presented at the International Stuttering Awareness Day Online Conference 2015, http://isad.isastutter.org/isad-2015/papers-presented-by-2015/research-therapy-and-support/the-importance-of-challenging-the-public-stigma-of-stuttering/

Butler, C. (2014). Wanted - straight talkers: Stammering and aesthetic labour. *Work, Employment & Society, 28*(5), 718-734.

Campbell, P. (2017). The way we talk. British Stammering Association (Last updated November 14th 2017), https://www.stammering.org/sites/default/files/waywetalk.pdf

Corrigan, P.W. & Watson, A.C. (2002). The paradox of self-stigma and mental illness. *Clinical Psychology: Science and Practice, 9*(1), 35-53.

Harvey, R. (2003). The sentence. In *When the Words Don't Come Out: Inside the Experience of Stammering*. London, UK: British Stammering Association.

Meredith, G. & Packman, A. (2015). The experiences of university students who stutter: A quantitative and qualitative study. *Procedia-Social and Behavioral Sciences, 193*, 318-319.

Mitchell, D. (2016). *Thirteen Ways of Looking at a Stammer*. Germany: Stotteren & Selbsthilfe Landesverband Ost e.V.

Mullin, E. (2016). Why Siri won't listen to millions of people with disabilities. *Scientific American*, https://www.scientificamerican.com/article/why-siri-won-t-listen-to-millions-of-people-with-disabilities/

Silverman, F.H. & Bongey, T.A. (1997). Nurses' attitudes toward physicians who stutter. *Fluency Disorder, 22*(1), 61-62.

St. Pierre, J. (2012). The construction of the disabled speaker: Locating stuttering in disability studies. *Canadian Journal of Disability Studies, 1*(3), 1-21.

Endnotes

[1] One could perhaps argue that in certain emergency situations fluent fast speech is needed for good healthcare. I would say, firstly, that these situations are surprisingly rare for most doctors and, secondly, I'm not sure I agree with it anyway – in my experience, calmness and clear-thinking under pressure are much more important qualities.

[2] Some people may argue that I am dismissing that stammering, as a physical act, is innately an undesirable activity, because it results in jaw pain, mouth tension and other negative sensations. This is a reasonable argument. However, I think these issues are most often insignificant compared to the profound effects of stigma against stammering on the lives of people who stammer. I am a person who stammers with a high degree of fluency, though, and perhaps not the right person to argue this.

[3] Perhaps particularly influenced by an individual's family beliefs and stigmas around stammering creating a unique social and environmental milieu that we each inhabit.

The big secret

Wendy Ronaldson

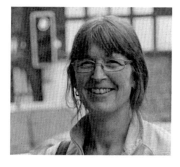

Visiting my son in Chester and out for a stroll round the lovely city centre.

The listener (Image 1)

I hate myself, frustrated and peeved off from hiding my stammer, I sit myself down in the art room. I am a self-employed domestic cleaner (a talk-free job), a DIY enthusiast, avid gardener, and a part-time artist – which I love. I open a drawer, grab some paper, no that's not good enough, I slide it back in place and rummage for heavier, smooth paper, that will do nicely. I choose heavier paper to work with so it will last longer, a bit like keeping the moment in suspense for longer. I lean over to a smaller drawer, pull it open and grab some colouring pencils. Being a covert stammerer was proving to be an issue. Although it had been an issue for a long time, I had begun to realize that I needed to seek help... me, seek help? Never!

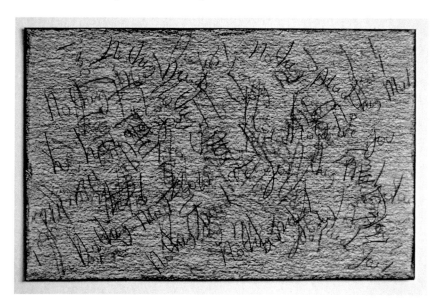

The listener (Image 1)

I had to endure bullying at school, or should I say, 'we'. I have an identical twin sister who also stammers; we were in most classes together along with breaks and lunchtimes. In class, we were mocked. Not just when we had to stand up and read out loud; any time my sister and I were together we were targets. I felt inferior, incapable of being able to do the basics of communication like everyone else. This led to the start of being covert. By covert I mean swapping stammered words for easy-to-speak words, forcing the words out or just keeping quiet. Anything to stop me from stammering and pulling a face. I am searching for my descriptions of stammered words. Stammered words are what I call repetition words: words I stammer on most of the time. Not always, though. This makes it more difficult for me because it's not consistent, so I wasn't in control of my speech and face pulling. Silent stammering is what I call blocks. My mouth takes shape to get the syllable out, but no sound comes out, losing the excitement of the conversation at that moment in time. A bit like wanting to laugh, but not being able to break a smile. At the age of 14, school for me was somewhere to avoid bullies whilst also trying to learn. Looking back, I now see school as an important part of childhood. I should have spoken out about the bullying, but threats to keep quiet were intense and ongoing, partly shaping my life for the future. School was like hurdles, up and down, never a flat race. It is where I made my best friends and worst enemies, making me stronger as a person inside. But this is where it stayed, inside. Those memories are ingrained after enduring mocking and bullying for five years, although the mocking did not stop after school.

At the time of this drawing, I was struggling to communicate. Years of avoiding speaking situations was taking its toll and I wanted to change my career and do the things I really wanted to do, not what my stammer was defining me to do. The fear of stammering for me had become overwhelming and shameful. I mustn't let it slip or they may laugh at me. Frustrated and emotional, I start to scribble words, using colour to define each different statement I use regularly; defining repetition. Nothing much. How are you? Nothing much. How are you? Nothing much. How are you? Wrapped tightly in a locked black box. That's all I ever seem to say, always switching the conversation over to the other person.

Earlier I had listened intently to a friend who had been away on holiday, telling me where and what they had been doing together. It all sounded very exciting. My holiday was described as 'Nothing much'. I went to Dunoon quite a lot. My husband is Scottish and his parents lived over there. I love it. Such a beautiful place, filled with lakes and twisty roads. Every time you turn a corner a lovely landscape waits to pop into view. Even though I wanted to brag about the beautiful countryside we had explored, I just stood there and said those two words. Nothing much. Feeling gutted, I thought, "You stupid cow."

The big secret (Image 2)

I love gardening. A form of recovery or a type of therapy? Two hundred and sixty feet of private space... and this is just the back garden; two sheds, a greenhouse and three lawns with flower borders. I spend time picking the flowers, planting bulbs, rearranging borders and generally making the place look beautiful. Just sitting and enjoying the space, watching the array of flowers and grasses in their various colours swaying in the wind. Delicate scents drifting up the garden path. A tree, picked from Lovers Lane in Scotland, majestically showing off its fresh green foliage. A canvas of colour in different medias and textures. I sit contemplating my inner self, scrutinizing my actions relating to my speech.

I pick up the pad and pencil and start drawing the garden shed. It won't be an ordinary shed: it will be huge and bulging with the conversations I wanted

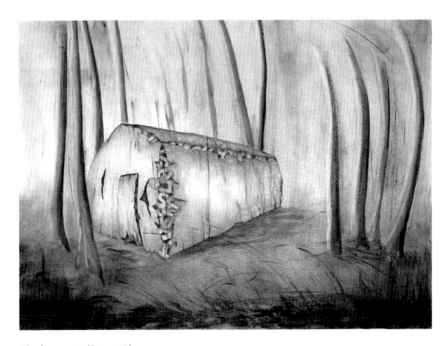

The big secret (Image 2)

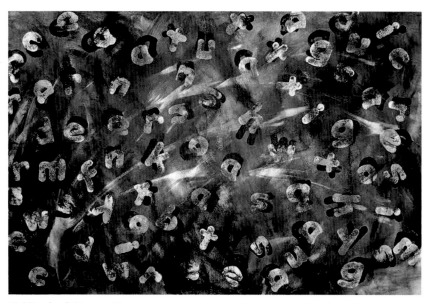

Holding back (Image 3)

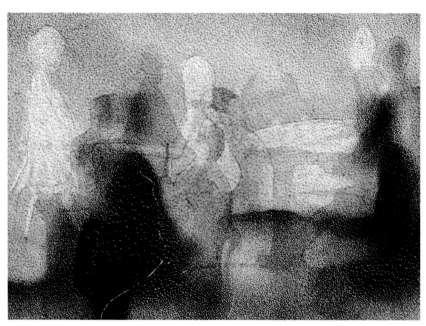

Conversation I (Image 4)

to tell people. But the door will be locked. I want to smash it down and let the words burst out. It's not about the aesthetics of the drawing; it's about saying more than that and capturing that feeling of reality, how it really is. I use a short piece of pastel stick to depict trees, which are bare and dissolve into the clouds, almost caressing, sheltering the shed, which is silently hidden away. I then rummage for a weakened mixture of ink and lay on a sweeping wash in the foreground. Adding colour doesn't feel right, so I pick up a graphite pencil. Again, using a fast sweeping action, I firmly lay marks for the grass, which has slowly been growing, left unattended and is now overgrown, festering. A feeling of relief overcomes me as the last blades of grass are depicted. The feeling of being trapped in a box and hidden away is now out in the open, but in visual form. Unable to talk about my issues at the time as it was too emotional, drawing gave me a different outlet for expression.

Holding back (Image 3)

My conversations were normally limited and short at the time of painting this piece. After not being able to ignore my stammer in a one-to-one conversation, a load of rubbish comes tumbling out from my tensed lips in the hope of staying fluent. I soon realized it was more important to say what you want to say and not be fluent - easier said than done though. Frustrated, with a large paintbrush in my hand, I eagerly stripped the white of the canvas. The heavy tension forced me to swipe on a flat colour, black, fast and furious, anything to rid the white expanse of space. This was then too heavy, so I dipped a brush in white paint and swiped on 3-4 shards of light. I then grabbed some letters, dipped them in paint and proceeded to build up the work. The letters are a collaboration of several words which represented my feelings at that moment in time, marked onto the silent canvas. After this piece of work was finished, I accepted that I needed to seek some help with my speech, and reluctantly booked to see a speech therapist.

Conversation I (Image 4)

My therapist was very patient with me in the beginning as I didn't communicate much. I just sat there and listened. I found it really difficult to be open with her, this person sitting straight across from me. As we sat face-to-face she was looking at me. I might pull a face if I spoke. This 'beginning' actually went on for around two years. Christine, my therapist, was very understanding and

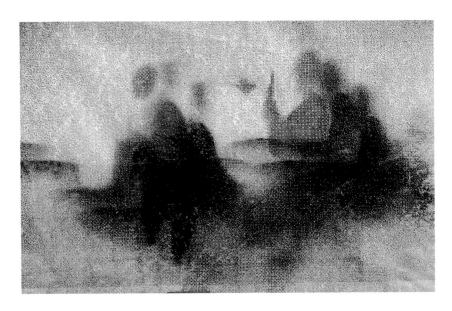

Conversation II (Image 5)

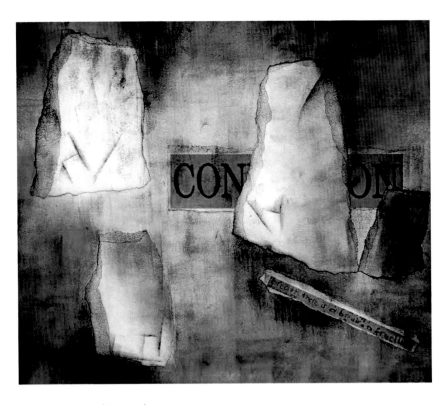

Maybe next time (Image 6)

explained the issues around stammering and the effects it causes. Eventually, I started to open up and accept my speech. It is who I am. I wanted to be me, not someone else. I worked on my communication skills with no cheating, no avoidance strategies… desensitizing and slowly becoming myself. For example, I struggled to pluck up the courage to call into a café and ask for a cappuccino. Cappuccino is not the easiest word to say when you have a stammer. It's my favourite drink, but I wouldn't normally ask for it for fear of stammering. Having avoided cafés for many years, I decided to portray communication visually. After grabbing some paper, I gently rubbed the background all over with graphite. Firstly, I wanted to include my absence, so I rubbed away my self-portrait, representing the times when I didn't feel able to communicate. I built up this process with colour and form using cut-outs of soaked pink newspaper, which were then transferred onto the work, portraying warmth and human flesh. Feeling the work was incomplete, I worked on a further layer to complete the depiction of window viewing; walking up to a café, looking through the window to see if it was busy, which it usually was, and then moving on. I transformed the images to represent distance and mystery as I always wondered what relationships these people had and what they were chatting about…

Conversation II (Image 5)

Feeling slightly more at ease with being overt, I again wanted to capture the connection of energy and spirit between human beings. Still window viewing, I conspicuously captured and memorized an interaction. The place was buzzing with people sharing each other's happenings over their favourite drinks or snacks. Back in the studio, I picked up a pencil and sketched from memory the interaction between two people conversing. I removed any unwanted distractions and discarded most of the colour, taking away the present and placing them in the past. I then stripped the figures of their sharp outlines, transforming them to forms of non-identity and giving the image a sense of distance leaving partly spirit and partly that present moment behind on the paper. A search for self-reflection on my past actions was emerging. Desensitization was becoming a lighter burden and more manageable.

Maybe next time (Image 6)

Although the burden was becoming lighter, I had just got back from speech therapy, frustrated again, "Neil," I shouted, "I am wasting the therapist's time.

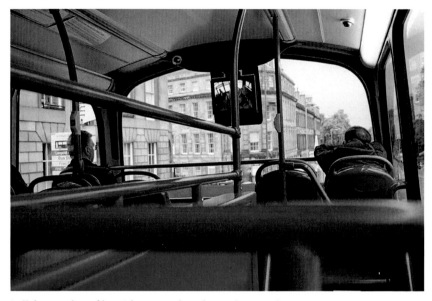

Still from a short film: *Silence speaks volumes* (Image 7)

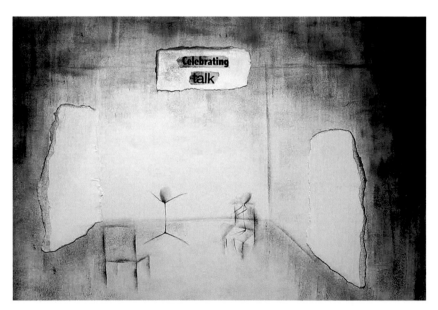

Celebrating talk (Image 8)

I didn't tell her anything." I wanted to, but I couldn't face it. She was looking at me and I thought I might stammer and pull a face.

The next weekend I went to an art exhibition at 20/21 Visual Arts Centre in Scunthorpe: 'We Are Not Alone'. It was based on taboo subjects. Viewers were invited to submit a piece of work, which could involve snippets of the works in the show. After photographing elements from several works of art, I spontaneously developed this piece of reflective work. The controlled tearing of forms represents moments in time which lead to somewhere different. Objects were added to these forms leaving out human elements, depicting absence. The colour shows promise, heading into a positive direction. I included text depicting covert and overt characteristics of stammering. Realizing it is OK to talk about issues and it does not need to be all 'hush hush' helps other people to understand they are not alone.

Still from a short film: Silence speaks volumes (Image 7)

Desensitizing my stammer through therapy has turned a corner. Although this work is ongoing, it has enabled me to begin the process of accepting myself for who I am. I decided to challenge myself and planned a fortnight in Edinburgh. Lots of places to see and things to do, but no car, so I had to travel on public transport. My husband joined me and we stayed at a relative's. The boys had different interests and did their own thing while I decided to jump on a bus and go exploring. My aim was to be overt. It didn't quite go to plan. A queue of people waiting behind me and the bus driver patiently waiting for my destination, so he could produce a ticket for me, was just a bit too much. The destination changed to a day saver ticket, which was easier to say. I had no idea where I was going and went and sat down. I sat at a window seat, hoping to spot my destination, but it didn't come into view. I restlessly got off the bus at an unknown destination in the middle of a housing estate. My destination was the Botanical Gardens and to find it now I had to ask a passer-by for directions. The still is from a short video of the start of my journey, depicting avoidance related to covert stammering. Even though progress is slow, I have moved on. Using public transport was something I avoided at that time but I got to my destination. The audio for the video had to be captured twice. Forty-five minutes talking into a microphone, hiding in the corner of a large room talking quietly with no expression or feeling, so no-one else could hear me. Taking on this challenge helped enormously with coming to terms with 'it is OK to be yourself'. Even though you are different you are still a human being and it doesn't matter *how* you say it, it is *what* you say that is important. Therapy and self-help groups have contributed to building communication skills, which is far more rewarding than being a covert stammerer.

Celebrating talk (Image 8)

The therapy room is depicted in this piece. Excitement and bold colours dominate. After a therapy session, I went straight into the studio at home and got out the coloured pencils, mountboard and pastels. I knew what I had to capture. The forms are still present, depicting moments in time which have changed size and shape to reflect the way I feel. Objects are now occupied with figures. One of these figures is my therapist, who is listening to me while I talk to her. The words flowed out through my lips with ease, like a butterfly dancing in the air. It never felt so good. Easy stammering, not plagued with tension. A feeling of connecting to me, my inner self. The colour, sharp and intense, represents happiness and joy, to me and to the viewer. During the chat I contained part of the excitement, which I depicted in this piece. Although I had the urge to jump up from the chair and dance, there was not enough room. I feel like a new person. The power of speech is enormous and carries many emotions. Embracing speech with a stammer for me has been a long journey, which has been built with knowledge, courage, perseverance and the love of other humans; embracing the need to engage and connect with them.

Keep kids talking: The impact of shame for children who stutter – A parent's perspective

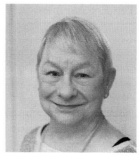

Standard boring mug shot!

Doreen (Dori) Lenz Holte

Increasing silence and disconnection permeate our memories of our son's childhood. These behaviours became a far greater burden than the stuttering he had struggled with since he was two-and-a-half. We had no clue that wanting a son who didn't stutter could lead to having a son who would rarely talk. Not talking was far easier and less shameful than failing to use the strategies he was learning and able to use so well in speech therapy. After six years of therapy, Eli went from a bubbly, chatty 3-year-old to a quiet, sullen, and depressed 9-year-old. When he was 10 he slumped into the chair next to me, and with tears running down his cheeks whispered, "I feel like I'm slipping into a dark hole. I just want to disappear." I took him on my lap, with his long legs dangling beyond mine and held him close. We cried together.

Dr Brené Brown (2007), licensed social worker and renowned author and speaker, states that:

> "Nothing silences us more effectively than shame... shame unravels our connection to others... In fact, I often refer to shame as the fear of disconnection – the fear of being perceived as flawed and unworthy of acceptance or belonging. Shame keeps us from telling our own stories and prevents us from listening to others tell their stories. We silence our voices and keep our secrets out of the fear of disconnection" (pp.267, 294).

Eli's shame around not being able to use his speech tools and techniques outside of the clinic setting was unravelling his connections to friends and family and to the world around him. It wasn't just his own struggle, but others' reactions to his struggle that contributed to this disconnection. His friends and brothers didn't seem to notice, but other kids laughed and teased and many adults stopped trying to engage Eli in conversation. I remember some adults tilting their head, forcing a fake smile, and freezing themselves in this position as Eli's cheeks turned bright red and he buried his chin in his shoulder and growled in order to say a word. It was uncomfortable for everyone and painful to watch.

Our early journey

Over a six-year period, we engaged five different speech therapists and drove hours each week to take Eli into the city for therapy. By the time he was 9, with the struggle as severe as ever, we felt out of options. During this time his diagnosis went from mild to moderate to severe. Yet, after most sessions, we were told how well he had done that day. I sat in on many sessions and knew he had no problem using his speech tools and techniques while in therapy – i.e., easy onsets, slow (turtle) talk, bouncing (Tigger talk), prolongations, stopping and starting over, taking a breath before talking, thinking about what he was going to say before he said it, etc. – but he refused to use them in real life. Why? Why would he choose to stutter, something he hated doing, when he could just use his tools instead?

When I expressed my frustration to the therapists about his unwillingness to use what he was learning, they encouraged me to keep practising with him at home. Was I doing something wrong during our practice sessions? Was I not doing practice time long enough or often enough or with enough patience or expertise? What level of focus would it take to make this go away? We were already driving him 45 minutes to an hour each way to attend speech therapy once or twice a week. I was already spending at least ten minutes to a half-hour five days a week sitting with him to practise his tools and techniques. They called it special time and, trust me, he didn't think it was very special.

The primary goal for Eli's early childhood therapy was fluency or, at best, less stuttering, and that was our goal too. For almost the entirety of his early childhood he heard messages that his speech was unacceptable and needed to be fixed. We cajoled and encouraged him to practise his techniques and, along with the speech therapists, applauded and rewarded him with stickers and candy when he did. I was confused and frustrated when he failed to use his techniques at home. We couldn't fathom a scenario where our beloved son would have to struggle with this for the rest of his life. It was simply unthinkable.

At 9 years of age, with his stuttering behaviour now so severe, we gave up on therapy and pretended to ignore his struggle, but of course it was all we thought about. We travelled to National Stuttering Association and FRIENDS conferences and found most attendees to be on board with the therapy their kids were receiving, although there was shared concern over the kids' refusal to use the tools and techniques. We came home confused and feeling at a complete loss. What we found was a seemingly undying support for the status quo – enlisting fluency shaping and stuttering modification strategies. The goal for fluency shaping is stutter-free speech by changing how you talk. The goal for stuttering modification is acceptance and less tension – by changing how you talk. All of Eli's therapy focused on changing how he talked, so in my mind these two strategies were one in the same. We were told these approaches were evidence-based and encouraged not to give up. I vacillated between wondering how much worse he'd be if we hadn't gone to therapy and a growing concern that the therapy may have done more harm than good.

Around this time we gained access to the Internet at home and I started to research and write – I suppose it was my way of feeling like at least I was doing something. Had we missed some important concept that was leading to our inability to embrace this therapy and make it work for Eli? Why did so many well-intentioned speech therapists persist in these approaches when they seemed to be failing so many of their young clients outside the clinic setting?

Exploring the research

Much to my surprise, I quickly uncovered other voices expressing concern about the most widely-accepted therapy approaches with children and the thin evidence that supported its popularity. Even more stunning to me was that those concerns were (and are) rarely, if ever, mentioned in the websites or print material of professional support organizations – the organizations parents first turn to for help. I pored through professional journals, published research, biographies and textbooks to gather what turned out to be the first body of work written by a parent, for parents, to reveal the uncertainties that underlie today's therapy for children who stutter. One of the most profound statements I came across was from Craig Coleman, Assistant Professor at Marshall University and Board-Certified Specialist in Fluency Disorders. Coleman (2015) states that:

> "We need to make quality of life the number one priority and the focus on reducing syllables stuttered is negatively impacting many children's quality of life well into adulthood...

> We sometimes pretend as a profession that with preschoolers
> we can treat them as if their stuttering is going to go away
> completely up until the point where it doesn't and then we
> can stop on a dime and say "just kidding, now it's okay to
> stutter – and we're going to successfully manage it." It's a
> dangerous trap that's hard to move away from when the kid
> turns 7 or 8 and is still stuttering."

The trap Coleman speaks of is set with two forms of bait: (1) that there is
evidence for these approaches, and (2) there is a 'window of opportunity' during
the preschool years when chances increase for therapy to result in recovery.

1 The evidence

The quality and integrity of the research used to justify the current treatments
for children is continually challenged by the researchers themselves. This isn't
surprising once one understands that there is little agreement as to how to define
stuttering or what the goals of research and therapy should be. A relatively
recent research study refers to high-quality evidence as being 'limited', with
'follow-up data needed', and 'surprisingly weak', with 'long-term effectiveness
unclear' (de Sonneville-Koedoot, Stolk, Rietveld, & Franken, 2015). Yet this
is the exact foundation that therapy for children is built upon.

Eighty percent of preschoolers will recover with or without therapy, and
to date there is no way to accurately predict which will persist (Månsson, 2000;
Yairi & Ambrose, 2005). The largest component of fluency shaping therapies
is instructing a child to change how they talk in order to not stutter (easy
onsets, smooth speech, taking a breath, using bounces, etc., ...). It is common
knowledge that this is something easily accomplished within the clinic setting,
but almost impossible to naturally carry over into the real world. With the
popular Lidcombe therapy, parents are trained to point out 'bumps' and praise
'smooth speech'. How many of these children pick up on the idea that their
bumpy speech is bad and smooth speech is good? How many of these kids
decide to choose silence rather than disappointing their adults or experiencing
a continual sense of failure?

My question is, what is the impact of these failed attempts on the children
who persist? These kinds of directives, over the years, have a tremendous
potential for increasing anxiety, shame, and disconnection and leaving this
population with a lifetime of unnecessary psychological and emotional

challenges that can limit their happiness and wellbeing. I do not think it can be worth the questionable gains that are made for the majority who will likely recover regardless.

A 2016 research study out of the University of Sheffield (Baxter et al., 2016) also sheds light on the overall quality of the research available today. Their study concluded that "two-thirds of the research studies around stuttering selected for the study were at a high risk of bias due to a number of issues including inadequate sample size, drop-out rate, inaccuracy, and selective reporting." The Sheffield study also speak to the limitations of the persistent use of the percent of syllables measurement outcomes:

> "... while measures of overt stuttering behaviours continue to dominate evaluation, the establishment of core outcomes which are of importance and relevance to people who stutter seems to be an urgent priority."

What core outcomes are most important to people who stutter? For too long we, as Eli's parents, believed that fluency was all that mattered. When we began to see our quest for fluency resulting in increased silence and withdrawal, we knew it was time to reassess our priorities. We had to change our desired outcome to keeping Eli talking and engaged in the world around him rather than reducing the stuttering behaviour.

2 The window of opportunity

The first time I heard about this 'window', Eli was 5 and the therapist told us that the 'window' was closing. She explained that the neuroplasticity in children's brains was more receptive to change until around 5. The image in my head was not just a closing window, but me frantically shoving Eli through the remaining sliver of an opening, as long as there was still an iota of hope to get him beyond this struggle. The therapist explained that we would start out with fluency-shaping techniques, and if that didn't work we would switch to stuttering modification techniques that would "make him stutter better" and in turn help him "accept his stutter and know it was okay to stutter". This all made sense, although I admit my heart sank a bit. I didn't want him to stutter better – I wanted him to not stutter at all. As long as that window had even a sliver of an opening, I wasn't giving up.

The 'window of opportunity' metaphor is still commonly conveyed by speech therapists to frantic parents, and fear of missing that window often results in an ill-informed rush to enlist professional support. I asked Dr Dennis Drayna, senior researcher with the National Institute on Deafness and Other Communication Disorders and former Stuttering Foundation Association board member, if there has been research that proves this 'window of opportunity' for young children exists. He said:

> "Actual evidence bearing on this in stuttering is surprisingly incomplete. A major obstacle here is that the changes that occur in the brain during stuttering recovery are difficult to see with existing technology."

The sense of urgency and panic often induced in parents by the closing window metaphor is unnecessary and unproductive, especially when there is no definitive evidence to support specific treatments and their impact on changes in the brain during this window. Most parents turn to the experts with a goal of getting their child fixed and this metaphor feeds into that desire. Therapists feel pressure to please the parents when often even they are not comfortable with that focus. Therapists must understand that parents can be educated.

Instead of dangling the 'window of opportunity' metaphor in front of parents, why not present them with Joseph Sheehan's (1970) iceberg theory. Sheehan's theory helps us to understand how observable speech behaviours labelled as stuttering are the tip of the iceberg, and blowing that tip off will do nothing to melt away the debilitating "fear, shame, guilt, anxiety, hopelessness, isolation, and denial" that can grow inside. The narrative around support for children must change. We must provide support that focuses on acceptance and nurturing that minimizes the psychological and emotional toll this struggle can have on a child's life. We must not risk exacerbating that toll with therapy that has fluency as its goal and sets too many children up to fail.

Although we were all told it really was okay for Eli to stutter, we didn't feel that way in our hearts and minds. The pressure to engage in therapy with a focus on making the behaviour stop contributed to the narrative that this was unwanted and unacceptable behaviour, for him, for us as his parents, and for society as a whole. As long as children who stutter and their parents are convinced by professional support organizations to engage in therapy focused on fixing the stutter or even 'managing' the behaviour, the lack of acceptance in society and the pain it generates will persist.

Continued stuttering = shame

Making Eli's speech the 'focus of everything' and using up so much of his childhood trying to attain fluency only led to silence and withdrawal. To him, controlling his stutter by using speech tools simply wasn't worth the effort. It was much easier to not talk. He wouldn't disappoint us, he wouldn't feel the shame and sense of failure because he didn't use his tools, and he wouldn't experience the pain and embarrassment of confused looks and having someone finish his sentence for him. Shame fuelled his growing silence. Psychologist Dr Michele Blume (2011) describes shame as:

> "... a silent killer... and a state where thought is inhibited and words are hard to find... and often results in an overwhelming impulse to hide or withdraw from social contact"

Eli didn't become increasingly silent because he stuttered. He became silent because he felt overwhelming shame around his stutter. How would this have played out if we had focused on minimizing shame rather than fixing the stutter? We'll never know, but from the time Eli was 3 until he was around 9, he was continually judged for his speech even when people were not intending to judge. Each successful therapy session increased expectations of success for all of us around his ability to talk without stuttering. Every week we struggled to hide our disappointment and frustration when his struggle continued and even worsened. He became increasingly sensitive to our reactions, and to this day he struggles more with us than with most others. This is what we risk when we expose our children to continual judgement around their speech – especially those children who persist in stuttering beyond the preschool years.

I can still see the 'once hopeful – now wounded' Eli sitting silently around the table or quickly giving up when someone talked over him. We spent so many years thinking the only thing we could do to protect him from rejection and humiliation was to find a cure for the stuttering. Our approach wasn't in any way protecting him. It wasn't just the silence and disengagement we observed – there was a sadness, a lack of confidence, a loss of exuberance for life, for playing, for living. We didn't realize how, in our minds, fluency had come to equal success, which meant stuttering equalled failure. The speech therapy he received as a young child was meant to make him more fluent and, in a way, it worked. When he didn't talk, he didn't stutter.

Developmentally inappropriate messages

The National Center on Birth Defects and Developmental Disabilities, Centers for Disease Control and Prevention reports the following developmental cognitive traits shared by children ages 6-10:

1 Have a strong desire to perform well and do things right.

2 Find criticism or failure difficult to handle.

3 View things as black and white, right or wrong, wonderful or terrible, with very little middle ground.

4 Naturally seek praise and want to conform.

We can better understand the risks of silence when an expectation of fluency is placed on these kids by putting those expectations in the context of these cognitive traits.

1 Have a strong desire to perform well and do things right. Children this age will go to great lengths to perform in a way they feel the adults in their lives think is 'right'. If they cannot talk 'right', it can easily feel safer to choose silence.

2 Find criticism or failure difficult to handle. Lack of applause, listeners who continually judge, reminders to use speech tools, even subtle reactions in a listener's face, are often interpreted as criticism and failure.

3 View things as black and white, right or wrong, wonderful or terrible, with very little middle ground. Applauding and rewarding when they use their speech tools or when they do not stutter and then telling them it's really okay to stutter isn't going to fly with this crowd. Cognitively speaking, they cannot manage those messages. Stuttering will be wrong and shameful if they have got the message that they can and should use speech tools to manage and/or control it.

4 Naturally seek praise and want to conform. Children conform because they naturally crave a strong sense of belonging in their family, their schools, their community. If they feel their stuttered speech is not conforming to the ways of the tribe and they cannot use the tools to fix their speech, then they will most likely feel shame and choose silence as the easiest way to conform and feel safe.

When Eli was 12, he told me, "I stopped talking as much because they said it was wrong." His talking was wrong – that's the message he came away with even though I witnessed him being told by therapists that it was okay to stutter. When I asked him if he remembered that, he frowned and said, "No." With his developmentally appropriate desire to do right, to conform, to please those around him, and to not experience a continual sense of failure, it was pretty unlikely, in the desperate roar of our enthusiastic praise and rewards for not stuttering, he would ever hear that it was really okay.

Cowboy therapy

Our lifeline came from an unlikely place – a horse ranch run by a quirky retired speech professor, Dr Jerry Halvorson. I remember my dramatic mindset shift when Dr Halvorson announced, "Our goal is to get Eli talking again because his previous therapy sucked all the fun right out of it." I was hearing the first thing that made sense to me on this entire journey.

Now instead of Eli being in therapy, it was Mom and Dad who were in therapy. As far as Eli was concerned, he was just helping some old cowboy with bad knees take care of his horses. During our visits to the ranch, Dr Halvorson role-modelled ways to get Eli talking again while together they mucked the horse stalls, fed the horses, and picked up rocks from the pasture. Through these get-togethers, we learned to not ask questions and instead to make statements that would likely generate unimpeded flow of conversation. We learned the importance of creating opportunities for Eli to be in charge, to build confidence, and to pursue his passions. We learned that different situations called for different kinds of listening. Dropping everything and zeroing in with eye contact every time he opened his mouth was adding unnecessary pressure. Although intense listening is occasionally appropriate, casual listening could work too. I came to realize that kids often explore their expanding world by babbling on and on and the more babble the better. We became adept at recreating scenarios when he talked more, stutter or no stutter, like when he was in the car, or with his friends, or fully engaged in an activity he loved. Within months his struggle started to melt away and over the years 'cowboy therapy' reversed the silence and disconnection and enabled the now 23-year-old Eli to flourish.

The narrative changed

Our lives had been shaped by a narrative around the need to fix our son. The problem wasn't with Eli's speech, it was with our perception of Eli's speech – as something that needed to be fixed. The therapy we accessed fully supported that perception and added layers of anxiety, like fuel to the fire, to his tension and struggle. Trekking to therapy once or twice a week, filling the tool box, and practising the use of those tools permeated our world. We felt pressure with each moment of stuttered speech, wondering which strategy would work best in that situation. We thought about how we should work on that strategy during special time and then wondered why he didn't use that strategy the next time he stuttered. We heard so many parents at conferences say (with a combination of hopefulness and exasperation), "He has his tool box, now he can use it when he wants to." All the tools are there, just open the box...

Cowboy therapy gave us a new narrative, and the shift in mindset was extraordinary. Now we celebrated his talking, noticed when talking was fun and came easily and recreated those environments as often as possible. We paid attention to his ever-changing interests and passions and made room for their exploration in his day. We role-modelled silliness, playfulness and imperfection by singing badly, dancing badly, and sharing our own failures as well as accomplishments. We learned to show our vulnerability so he would feel comfortable showing his. We learned that it was far more important to raise a happy, well-rounded, productive and confident child than a child who doesn't stutter.

We need our kids to understand that stuttering is in no way equal to failure. Too much of the narrative around stuttering and the focus on fixing the behaviour is setting our children up for a lifetime of unnecessary struggle that permeates the entirety of their long-term wellbeing. Author and person who stammers, Cameron Raynes, shares his experience with coming to realize the impact his internal narrative was having over his life:

> "My definition of a good day used to be, 'A good day is one where I don't stutter, especially in front of a stranger', which was kind of pathetic and sad. I decided the only way forward was to take that definition and turn it upside down. My new definition became – 'A good day is one where I do stutter, especially in front of a stranger.'"

The narratives needs to change – for parents, for speech therapists, for researchers, for the children themselves and for society as a whole. This can only happen when we shift away from the goal of eliminating or reducing the percent of syllables stuttered.

The research study, referred to earlier, that continually pointed out the shortcomings of previous research was comparing an indirect therapy that focuses on modifying the child's environment to facilitate easier speech (RESTART -Demands and Capacities Model) with a direct operant conditioning therapy (Lidcombe). The researchers concluded that they successfully proved that either of these two therapies were better than no therapy at all. At the same time, they were quick to point out that these are two very (very) different therapies. They acknowledged that the common components of increased one-on-one time with parents, the reduction of linguistic demands, and an increase in emotional support were likely to have had the greatest impact (de Sonneville-Koedoot et al., 2015).

The narratives children adopt are greatly shaped by their parents' narratives and that's where therapy needs to start. We need to develop safe and effective support focused on parents and driven by outcomes that include maintaining or increasing level of a child's verbal output, overall confidence, feeling of empowerment, and their engagement in the world around them.

Recently we were sitting around the kitchen table with our two older sons (not Eli) and some of their friends. Their friends were talking about how quiet our one son was and he said, "Hey, Abe [his twin] is the really quiet one, I'm next, and then Eli – he's the extrovert!" It never dawned on me – but that is the absolute truth. Why hadn't I noticed this before? Did my own internal narrative and ingrained stereotypes blind me to the fact that out of my three children, the one who stuttered grew up to be the most outgoing and extroverted? I am so grateful that we got him back! I want to end with Eli's words from a recent essay he wrote:

> "A facet of my life that has had an undeniable impact on who I am now is my struggle with my stutter. As far as my memory goes back I have had a speech impediment that, at times, rendered me emotionally and physically exhausted. As a very young child I took part in speech therapy that backfired spectacularly. As a result when I was seven years old I found that the best way to not stutter was to not talk and for a couple years I retreated into myself and spoke only when necessary. This is not who I am today. Since those quiet years, with the help of a retired speech language pathologist and my amazing family and friends, I learned to be comfortable with my voice and embrace the feeling of stepping outside of my comfort zone. Coming out of those years I learned something that is vitally important to how I live: Giving up is always an option. Every day I can choose to not talk and every day I can choose to not pursue my ambitions. What drives my life is that I don't."

Go to www.voiceunearthed.com to get updates on Eli and for the Voice Unearthed Blog, Vlog, member stories and more. *Voice Unearthed: Hope, Help, and a Wake-Up Call* is available at Amazon.com. Also join us in the Voice Unearthed Facebook Group – the largest parent support group in the world for children who stutter.

References

Baxter, S., Johnson, M., Blank, L., Cantrell, A., Brumfitt, S., Enderby, P., & Goyder, E. (2016). Non-pharmacological interventions for stuttering in children and adults: A systematic review and evaluation of clinical effectiveness, and exploration of barrier to successful outcomes. *Health Technology Assessment, 20*(2), 1–302.

Blume, M.L. (2011). Understanding and working through shame in therapy. Retrieved from http://drmicheleblume.com/understanding-and-working-through-shame-in-therapy/

Brown, B. (2007). *I Thought it was Just Me [But it Wasn't]*. New York, NY: Gotham Books.

Coleman, C. & Reitzes, P. (2015). Is there a best stuttering treatment? *StutterTalk, 494* (February 10, 2015).

de Sonneville-Koedoot, C., Stolk, E., Rietveld, T., & Franken, M.-C. (2015). Direct versus indirect treatment for preschool children who stutter: The RESTART randomized trial. *PloS One, 10*(7), e0133758.

Månsson, H. (2000). Childhood stuttering: Incidence and development. *Journal of Fluency Disorders, 25*(1), 47–57.

Sheehan, J.G. (1970). *Stuttering: Research and Therapy*. New York: Harper & Row.

Yairi, E. & Ambrose, N. (2005). *Early Childhood Stuttering for Clinicians by Clinicians*. Austin, TX: Pro-Ed.

On stuttering activism and resistance

Zahari Richter

I am writing this chapter to make an important distinction between 'activism' and 'resistance' as two separate types of responses to disability oppression. Stuttering social activism and resistance have been defined by their practitioners, on the fly, to explain efforts taken to deal with either the neglect or repression of disabled experience. Activism is a coordinated and collective strategy of institutional challenge. Resistance represents opposition to institutional involvement and can be accomplished individually. I make the distinction in order to highlight that, depending on an individual's experiences and framings, either activism or resistance may be justified.

My father was a stuttering activist. He ran a support group for six to eight people with speech impediments in the mid-1980s in Miami, Florida. His organization existed purely for the goal of social support. While he was connected to an early iteration of the National Stuttering Association, his organization dealt heavily with the anxiety of being a stutterer in a smooth-speaking world. My father's activism was connected to his own profession of social worker. His small group sought greater social and professional resources. This was based on alignment with major institutional forces that had already targeted stuttering for assimilation within a caring-professions model.

I am a resistor. My role in stuttering organizing, as someone committed to resistance, reflects my experiences as a victim of repression on the basis of my speech difference. I distinguish my work as a writer and organizer of the independent blogging website DidIStutter.org as fundamentally distinct from the work of my father and the tasks of the National Stuttering Association. My work at DidIStutter.org is resistance: criticizing the ideology of speech-language pathology and responding to the harms initiated by its routine interventions into the lives of young people with speech impediments.

Resistance culminates in refusal, in energy turned against itself. Resistance always means principled opposition and clear boundaries and goals that are being overridden in the current day. Resistance is risky; you gain no friends when you expose the dystopic elements of society. I have lost many friends from my desire to expose the truth of the world.

The perils of activism

Activism has as many costs as benefits. The word 'activism' was coined from a group advocating for Sweden to become involved in World War I but it also has an etymological association with direct action. Therefore, both explicitly and implicitly, the word 'activism' carries the meaning of pleading for institutional action into a given problem. Originally, the institution-of-action was the state, but in recent times the state has spread its resources out and the institutions that people ask to act are corporate as well. Activism has as many downsides as it does benefit in the case of taking action to ameliorate social problems.

Stuttering activism has been dominated by what is called the stuttering self-help movement. I view the self-help movement as achieving much in terms of uniting stutterers and causing people with speech impairments to think more critically about their social devaluation. My own critical consciousness about stuttering is after all an outgrowth of my father's participation in the stuttering self-help movement. But there is a validity to theories which suggest even organizations and movements with the best of intentions can degrade in their attachment to their original principles. As I will argue in the next paragraph, I believe this fate has befallen the stuttering self-help movement.

Stuttering self-help activists, over the years, have become more and more closely aligned with the clinical practitioners of speech language pathology. To assume that this was not intended would be a mistake. The National Stuttering Association declares its mission to be "a catalyst for research into effective treatment for stuttering while encouraging the search for its cause and cure". The search for a cause and cure to stuttering is obviously a goal that requires begging for more money to be filtered into privately-run clinics and state-funded posts devoted to speech language pathology. The search for a cause and cure does not defend stuttering people against the major changes to their lives that would be initiated by such a cure, nor does it support the need of stuttering people not to be traumatized by having their speech differences stigmatized. Approaching stuttering solely on an individual level and without consideration of social technologies and social design is an inherently reactionary approach to stuttering politics. To invest so much time and effort into correcting a body is to give up a greater and more profound opportunity: to redesign society to make stuttering fit easier into the spoken fabric. I believe 'stuttering self-help' as a concept has much possibility, but we must help ourselves not to be corrected; rather to build a society where our vocal tics are less irruptive and are more welcomed by the conversational environment.

Damaging medicalisation

I practise resistance in response to the very specific unkind intrusion of speech therapists in my own life. If I felt abused by speech therapy then others are also likely to have experienced mental angst from the intrusion of speech-language pathologists (SLPs). The magnitude of medical harm from speech pathology requires that we act immediately to reduce routine speech therapy for children and adults who stammer.

My experiences of speech language pathology within school are the source of my opposition to treatment and cure. While in elementary school, I was repeatedly brought inside a speech pathologist's office, where I remember being convinced and coerced to speak more slowly and in a sing-songy manner. Prior to meeting the speech therapist at the age of 8 in the third-grade, I had only ever noticed my own stutter when school children remarked on it in a disparaging manner. To meet a professional whose entire goal and effort happened to align entirely with the agenda of schoolyard bullies was a shock to me at 8 and 9 – just as it is a shock to me now. As a young person, I refused to speak in the slow but sing-songy way that the speech therapist taught me to avoid repeating words or syllables. Even at that age I had felt I was being taught to fake who I was.

If speech language pathology is the intervention that stuttering activists seek from the government, medicine and private sphere, there is at least a conversation to be had about its medical necessity. While many medical fields seek to fix obviously painful maladies, the repetition of syllables is not inherently risky to health. If clinical speech pathology must bring up talk of 'secondary impairments' even to justify the study of stuttering cure in the first place, it becomes elaborately clear to me that the stutter itself is not the problem. If anxiety is a secondary impairment from stuttering, let stutterers perhaps receive extra priority for psychotherapy. If there are physical problems that emerge in jaws that do stutter, let that problem too be managed by someone that specializes in the study of jaw or throat ailments. The stutter itself is only a negative bodily development if making people occasionally wait an extra two to ten minutes is a pathological emergency. This is all just to say, the burden should be on speech pathologists to prove their legitimacy on something more than merely auditory aesthetics.

The origins of resistance at DidIStutter.org

Instead of seeking institutional intervention from a form of knowledge whose apex is the maintenance of an implicit norm, I resist the compulsion to stem stuttering and instead challenge all parts of smooth-speaking society to be more welcoming and receptive to stuttering people. I blame clinical speech language pathology for failing to question ideological devaluations of stuttering present in economics, religion and other long-standing social institutions. Indeed, in economics, the stutter interrupts the social and professional expectations of smooth and efficient speech; this can directly limit the stutterer's ability to find work. In religion, stuttering is sometimes treated either as a sign of divinity or a curse for sins or negative character. In politics or democracy, stutterers may be prevented from holding political power because they do not meet normative expectations of refined speech.

I, and my work in disability-organizing as part of DidIStutter.org, am connected to a disability rights movement that has offered vibrant new ways of resisting institutions and merciless workplaces in the form of accessibility and accommodations enforced by laws. In the 1970s and 1980s, the US disability rights movement was very successful in organizing (a semblance of) unity between disability activists coming from different impairment communities to use direct action to demand access to public space and institutions as well as accommodations in schools. The victories of these movements were not comprehensive: accessibility regulations are not easy to enforce without exhaustive, rarely successful court cases and the work has not guaranteed people with disabilities equal employment.

These rights have not yet extended to stutterers. Primarily, stuttering and other speech impairments are too complex and nuanced to consider with mental or physical disability categories. Unlike many other impairments, accessibility for stutterers is abstract. There are no ramps that can be installed which will make stutterers more present in conversations. Access for stutterers requires imagining accessibility in completely distinct terms from the physical technologies that are most often used to offer access.

The current pathologization of stammering comes both from an obsession with human speech as an expression of inner consciousness and from a pre-digital and pre-multimedia technological epoch where speech is expected to go on without enhancement. The use of alternative devices, such as text-to-speech (also known to autistics as an 'interaction board') or the adaptation of other literacies, such as sign language, can offer a way to extend the mediums offered to voice without conditioning the mind to feel its voice is inadequate. As a child, I only ever considered speech therapy when I felt extremely belittled by people who chose to give my speech less patience, time and effort. Without the onslaught of disablist shaming of stutterers and with the thoughtful use of adjustments in society for people who stammer, the entire reason for speech pathology fades.

My father's own experiences as a stuttering activist, like mine as a stuttering resistor, come from the experience of prejudice and discrimination against disability. As I was growing up, my father repeatedly recalled being mocked by parents, schoolyard peers, and even teachers and bosses. My father spent much of his life in great mental anguish over the continued disapproval and enmity that he experienced in being a stutterer in a smooth-speaking society. I have come to my viewpoints and positions in part as a result of being his child and being raised by him to feel empowered about my speech and not to feel devalued by family members, students, speech language pathologists, or other superiors. With my father, I dream of a day when all stutterers are taught that there is nothing wrong with them and that it does not matter how long it takes you to say a word or how many misunderstandings you have in daily conversations and to instead realize that what matters is the effort you put in and the spirit in your everyday expressions.

Patrick Campbell: A friend who stammers took this photo of me in Amsterdam after a stammering youth meeting in Holland in 2014; it is my go to photo to this day.

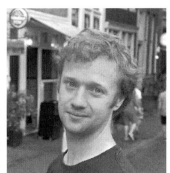

Ann Packman: That persistent Julius Sumner Miller question, "Why is it so?"

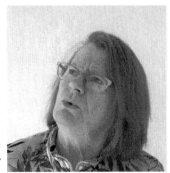

Grant Meredith: Stuttering sage and freedom of speech warrior

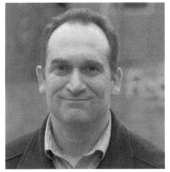

Coming together in collaboration: Elephants, canyons and umbrellas in the stuttering community

Patrick Campbell in conversation with Ann Packman and Grant Meredith

The social model and its theoretical offshoots, such as stuttering pride, offer the chance to transform both society's and our own view of stuttering. But, at the same time, they could, and indeed have, proved divisive within the stuttering community. Vicious arguments have erupted, particularly in online forums. Some people who stutter cannot fathom the idea of having pride associated with what they see as a deficit that needs to be eliminated.

I can feel this divisiveness in myself. I am becoming drawn towards a social model perspective. Its personal role in empowering my own voice encourages me to be evangelical about the larger role it should have in stuttering therapy and society. I feel myself being internally critical of those taking up alternate positions. Yet, I believe individual choice needs to be respected. The great majority of those aligned with the medical model of stuttering wish to help those who stutter as much as I do – just with different approaches.

The sweeping wave of partisanship in Western politics, that leaves less and less room for considered, moderate positions, perhaps offers a worrying harbinger for stuttering. I fear we will be left with a situation where therapists and people who stutter have to choose sides when in reality we are all on the same team for a rarely respected speech difference.

Disturbingly, perhaps we can already see the beginnings of divisions in our own community. Here in the UK, there is a tension developing between those who follow an acceptance and pride-based approach to their stammer whilst others continue to work towards a way to control, or even potentially to cure, their stammer. Are feuds and divisions unavoidable within our community?

To look into how we can ensure fruitful and productive teamwork between individuals and organizations coming from vastly differing experiences of stuttering, I spoke with Grant Meredith and Ann Packman. Their verbatim quotes from this discussion go alongside the text at appropriate moments to help lend context and meaning.

Background

To me, Grant and Ann hold very different theoretical perspectives. Ann, on the face of it, appears medical model-orientated. She has been involved in the development of fluency improving speech techniques like the Lidcombe and Camperdown programs; programs that try to fix stuttered speech for children and adults, respectively. Grant, on the other hand, has grown up as a person who stutters. He describes it as "a shaping experience" and a "characteristic". He had a strong, supportive childhood in an environment that accepted his speech; in turn, Grant is comfortable with his own stutter. He has become an academic in his own right and he is the leader of the Technologies for Empowering People for Participation in Society (TEPPS) Programme.

You could see the potential for disagreements. Ann looking into fluency treatments for stuttering; Grant proudly living his life with his stutter as a university lecturer. However, they have seen each other as complementary since their collaboration began.

Grant feels that this cross-collaboration allows his research to go into areas rarely explored in stuttering: to ask questions others are afraid to ask or simply do not consider. Ann sees Grant as a voice of a person who stutters within the academic sphere. The energy that comes from this viewpoint and his different ways of thinking could bring new insights to stuttering therapy and her own research.

I was surprised and pleased to hear of their successful collaboration from such differing viewpoints. It left me wondering whether all issues are reconcilable with considered debate or whether there are some (maybe unspoken) wedge issues in stuttering therapy that do fundamentally divide the stuttering community.

Ann: I trained as a speech pathologist many, many years ago. My main work is with people who stutter as a teacher, researcher and therapist. I work in Australia at the University of Technology Sydney. I have an interest in all aspects of stuttering and its treatments. I'm a bit of a theorist... so I enjoy investigating the cause and nature of stuttering. I am particularly interested in the issues students who stutter have at school.

Grant: I am a person who stutters of course. I'm a lecturer and academic at the Federation University Australia and I'm an Associate Dean of Student Retention and Success. So, my job is to keep students motivated and s-s-supported and hopefully have very successful outcomes. My research is mainly IT r-related... It is looking at assertive t-t-t-technologies to aid people with special needs to contribute more to s-s-society. I am also studying for a PhD, looking at the university experiences of students who stutter.

Grant: It isn't illegal to stutter, you know.

Grant: We come up with questions or ideas that are very out of the box. It's almost a sense of erm f-freedom we b-b-both bring we both bring. Ann is highly esteemed... obviously, very scientific. I bring my IT knowledge and stuff too, so we actually complement each. We have freedom to actually ask questions and to explore areas others haven't looked at much. Consequently, Ann and I have several published journal articles together and also presented co-authored papers at conferences. One of which was on stuttering's position as a disability in Rome six years ago: "Is Stuttering a Disability?"

Ann: Doing research would mean Grant would bring his own experience to his research area. Rather than me just hearing it as a researcher or speech pathologist. Here was someone wanting to research stuttering, but who had that personal experience to bring to his research.

Blind men and an elephant: Social anxiety in stuttering

There's a famous Indian parable about blind men coming upon an elephant for the first time[1]. Each blind man investigates a different part of the elephant. Each comes to a different conclusion as to the animal in front of him based on his own limited perspective of the situation: one feels its trunk and thinks that the animal is a snake, another reaches for its legs and thinks it is a tree trunk, and another its side and thinks it is a wall. Stuttering has the potential to be a similar experience. We all experience a different perspective of stuttering: to begin with, no two stutters are alike and we each, as individuals, inhabit our own unique social milieu. These differing perspectives of stuttering, generated through individual experience, can lead us to different understandings of its nature. I feel this is particularly salient in stuttering-related social anxiety research.

Social anxiety has become a hot topic in stuttering research. Social anxiety is a medical diagnosis of increased anxiety in social situations that prevents an individual from interacting in a 'normal' fashion. Ann, as part of her role in the team at the Australian Stuttering Research Centre in Sydney, is an expert on social anxiety in people who stutter and has researched it for many years from a medical perspective. This work has identified that a high number of people who stutter meet the diagnostic criteria for social anxiety. It has also developed treatments targeted at reducing social anxiety in people who stutter and begun to look at its root cause.

If I were to talk about similar negative emotions in the context of stuttering – fear of speaking, fear of being identified as different – I would draw upon public stigma in society and the consequent process of internalization that can lead to self-stigma. I would see people who stutter as having a natural reaction of anxiety to the hostile society around them, rather than a medical diagnosis. I understand social anxiety in stuttering through my social model lens of life as a person who stutter, just as Ann reaches for her medical model as a therapist.

---

1 This is a surprisingly oft-used allegory in stuttering. Its first use is traceable to Wendell Johnson in 1958.

Ann: Social anxiety is much more prevalent in adults who stutter. Social anxiety is a fear of speaking in social situations. Technically, it is fear of negative evaluation... some example quotes I have heard [from people who stutter]: 'no-one will like me if I stutter', 'people won't believe what I say'. So, we have designed a cognitive behavioral therapy program specifically for people who stutter.

Ann: I think [social anxiety arises] because of external, or even family relations, teasing, bullying, made to feel inferior at school, sometimes even at home... So yes, I think people come to think of themselves that way. That would be my view.

But really, are Ann and I that far apart in our understandings of this phenomenon in people who stutter?

In conversation, we each gravitate to similar underlying issues, just from different points of view. I agree with a lot of what Ann says. Ann, through her Centre's research, under the medical lens has dissected the source of this social anxiety and traces it back to childhood bullying. She's targeting interventions to change the atmosphere of school to help people who stutter, in particular to make the environment less hostile (and references and uses the social model in talks). Our viewpoints and overall aims align well.

So perhaps we can consider the social model and the medical model, in the case of social anxiety, are beginning to get a feel for a larger picture and come together in a joint understanding. We aren't having a divisive disagreement over social anxiety as an issue for people who stutter. We are just understanding different parts of the issue, this stuttering elephant.

Ann: *I think teachers are really the clue here and, Grant, you have a great experience... If teachers can be aware of this [bullying about stuttering]. And do more to stop this happening. That would be a big step for building confidence and courage.*

Ann: *As a result, each year I lead a forum for final year university teaching students in which we (researchers, therapists, and people who stutter) talk to soon-to-be teachers about stuttering and how teachers can support students who stutter in the classroom... We use the social model in these sessions to help teachers better understand how they can get the children to engage.*

Canyons in the stuttering community

A canyon is a deep cleft that exists between two cliffs. It is not possible to cross from one side of a canyon to the other without great effort. You have to choose which side of the canyon you stand on. I think canyons, as well as elephants, exist in stuttering.

The example I wish to use is a continual flashpoint of debate in the stuttering community. It is whether therapy aimed to make children who stutter fluent is the best option for children who stutter.

To me, you have to stand on one side of this debate. We are not understanding the same issues from different perspectives; we are taking fundamental positions on a challenging topic.

The medical model tries to cure the 'defect' seemingly at the heart of the disorder – in this case, making people who stutter become fluent. In stuttering, medical studies have shown that fluency-based therapy programmes improve the 'recovery' rates of children who stutter. The exact improvement in 'recovery' rates, what 'recovery' from stuttering looks like, and the best therapy to facilitate this remain in dispute, but the evidence does support an improvement in return to natural fluency if children are placed in a fluency-oriented treatment programme at a young age.

This leaves therapists coming from a medical model point of view only one position to take: to advocate for fluency-based therapy. If a child who stutters gains more fluency then their disability is alleviated. If a child who stutters becomes completely fluent then the disability disappears completely. The logic is compelling and commonplace in a society that largely upholds the medical model of disability as the dominant narrative around difference.

Patrick: *I have a question for you, Ann. Would you say every child who stammers needs therapy?*

Ann: *Talking about preschoolers, when they start stuttering... well, I do think it's a choice of the parent. I would say yes. I think so, yes. But if a parent does not want speech therapy that's of course their decision. You know there's some discussion of the effectiveness of early intervention – let's call it that – even if it doesn't take the stuttering away, it appears in every child to reduce it a lot, maybe that's a good thing. That would be my view.*

A social model perspective leads to a different view on stuttering therapy for children. The social model places the burden of disability on an ill-conceived society. Therapy, from a social model perspective, would be for society to ensure an environment in which the stuttering child is not disadvantaged. Social model therapy for stuttering would likely involve talking to parents about how to best create a supportive environment for children who stutter and education for a child's school on stuttering. The mainstay of therapy would not be fluency.

However, there are subtleties. The social model makes a distinction between disability and impairment. It does not necessarily see improving impairments through the medical model as wrong. Some people who stutter experience physical jaw pain when they speak and have intense struggle – the social model would support treatment of the stuttering itself to help alleviate these issues. Fluency-based therapy is therefore possible working from a social model framework, perhaps even encouraged, but it gets tricky.

Issues develop when treating impairments creates stigma for the disorder: when you try to treat the impairment for some, you exacerbate the disability for others. I can see the potential for this in stuttering therapy. Lidcombe therapy encourages parents to make subtle interventions and statements on their child's speech. For example, a piece of stuttered speech might be met with "that was bumpy, why not try it again?" Perhaps not directly stigmatizing, but statements like this risk further deepening the sense that stuttering is wrong to a young child, and thus exacerbate its potential to disable in later life when they view their own speech as abnormal.

For this reason, I see a social model perspective as being irreconcilable with many fluency-based therapies in use today that either explicitly or implicitly discourage stuttered speech.

Patrick: *Surely, if you truly want change for people who stammer you have got to be prepared for people who stutter to just stammer and not try to bend to society's wants of fluency?*

Grant: *If I had a child who started to stutter would I seek treatment for that child? I would say yes, I would personally, because of my knowledge of the evidence that intervention into children as early as possible improves the outcomes for them being fluent... Because I have seen the journeys of so many people who stammer which have been negative and I don't mind giving my child the opportunity not to stutter.*

Emerging models of disability (to my mind at least) can lead to an even more extreme, almost hostile viewpoint on fluency-based stuttering therapy. In the political/relational model, stuttering can become understood as a form of natural human diversity. A child who stutters is simply communicating with a unique voice. To try to eradicate their way of speaking would be immoral.

A similar viewpoint is being taken by some within the neurodiversity movement in Autism. Autism is classically treated with applied behaviour analysis, that tries to get rid of 'odd' behaviours which can make it difficult to fit in to normal society. In these therapies, significant efforts are made to encourage appropriate eye contact and remove autistic tics. However, some in the neurodiversity movement are now questioning the appropriateness of this behaviour training. Are these tics and behaviours just part of the autistic aesthetic? Are they natural signs that the person belongs to a unique tribe of individuals?

A similar argument could be put forward for the treatment of children who stutter with fluency-based therapies. Are you taking away a fundamental part of their aesthetic, their unique identity, without their consent?

Of course, these models are imperfect attempts to capture a system of thought. None of us aligns perfectly to an individual model in our views and opinions on stuttering in real life.

Indeed, Grant goes for the jugular when we discuss the issue in real life. He loads the situation with parental responsibility and feeling. It changes the question's dynamic. Suddenly, the necessary pragmatism needed to succeed in the real, gritty, topsy-turvy, capitalist world comes into play: the hypothetical models with utopian ideals can fall by the wayside. We all want the best for those connected to us. What does it matter being a bit of hypocrite if it gives your child the best start in life?

Nevertheless (as someone who has not got children) I stand firm on my academic ramblings. I have to, else I would publicly be left in that hypocritical abyss of the canyon. I do believe, ultimately, we each have to choose a side of this stuttering canyon: whether fluency-based therapy helps or hinders children who stutter.

Grant: *Patrick, I have question for you, Patrick, erm, in the not too distant future you and your partner will have a child.*

Patrick: *That's fairly distant at the moment... anyway*

Grant: *You are a handsome man, Patrick... Let's say your child develops a stutter, but you do provide a good holistic environment you know. How would you answer your child when your child is sixteen, perhaps they have experienced some negative stigma and some problems and they ask, "Dad, why did you not intervene?"*

Patrick: *I think what I would say back erm if we don't have people who stutter proudly being people who stammer then we will never change anything around stuttering. So, I think even offering fluency-based therapy to him I would be implying it would be a negative to stammer and just propagating society's negative views of stammering. I wouldn't be helping the larger problem in society [stigma against people who stammer].*

The umbrella: Equality for people who stutter

Whilst there may be many potential areas of disagreement in the stuttering community, there are some areas on which we can nearly all agree. These issues can ensure we stay together, under their umbrella, to fight for a unifying cause. The most pressing of these, to me, is equality for people who stutter.

We live in a society that is prejudiced against people who stutter, which can prevent them from achieving everything they want to in life. Research has shown people who stutter are generally seen as 'weaker', 'less confident' and 'less able' than fluent people. Kenneth St. Louis made a good chronicle of this in his book, *Stuttering Meets Stereotype, Stigma and Discrimination*. This prejudice has real-life consequences across all stages of life:

- Children who stutter are more likely to be bullied in school

- People who stutter are at higher risk of mental health problems than the general population

- People who stutter can be excluded from employment and may find it more challenging to get a job.

I have experienced these issues in my own life and I am sure many readers have as well. The 'canyons' which may exist within the stuttering community are trifling compared to the issue of daily prejudice and discrimination against stuttering which affects the lives of nearly all people who stutter.

As spoken about in depth in Michael Boyle's chapter, there are many different ways to challenge the public stigma related to stuttering. Stuttering Pride is perhaps a strong response to public stigma, but there are others, such as educational approaches from professionals. These can work in tandem and are not mutually exclusive.

The same is true for the stuttering community. We can work in tandem, like Grant and Ann. We may debate our differences but we must ensure we work together towards the aim of making society a better place for all people who stutter.

Recommended further reading and references

Craig, A. & Tran, Y. (2005, May 1). What is the relationship between stuttering and anxiety? British Stuttering Association Website. Retrieved February 12th, 2019, https://www.stammering.org/speaking-out/articles/what-relationship-between-stuttering-and-anxiety

Harmon, A. (2004, December 20). How about not 'curing' us, some Autistics are pleading. *The New Yorker*. Retrieved February 12th, 2019, from https://www.nytimes.com/2004/12/20/health/how-about-not-curing-us-some-autistics-are-pleading.html

Meredith, G. (2016, October 1). Fostering a culture of pride. International Stuttering Awareness Day Online Conference. Retrieved February 12th, 2019, http://isad.isastutter.org/isad-2016/papers-presented-by-2016/stories-and-experiences-with-stuttering-by-pws/fostering-a-culture-of-pride-grant-meredith/

Meredith, G. & Harrison, T. (2014, October 1). Acceptance and the rise of pride. International Stuttering Awareness Day Online Conference. Retrieved February 12th, 2019, http://isad.isastutter.org/isad-2014/papers-presented-by/perceptions-and-interpretations/acceptance-and-the-rise-of-pride/

Packman, A. & Meredith, G. (2012). Is Stuttering a Disability? In *Proceedings of the International Conference on Stuttering*, Rome.

St. Louis, K. (2015). *Stuttering Meets Stereotype, Stigma, and Discrimination: An Overview of Attitude Research*. West Virginia: West Virginia University Press

Making change happen: How we can work together to decrease stigma

Michael P. Boyle

Introduction

In this chapter I hope to inform you about the different roles of professionals and advocates in challenging the public stigma associated with stuttering. There are different agendas, processes, and goals for reducing the stigma faced by people who stutter (PWS), and sometimes these differences can lead to conflict between advocates and professionals. I have an interest in this topic because I have personally seen divisions that can occur between professionals and advocates. For example, many caring professionals who dedicate their lives to helping PWS can become upset when they hear advocates state that speech therapy should not be recommended for PWS. On the other hand, advocates can become upset when professionals claim to know what is best for them and attempt to change them. Seeing debates between professionals and advocates in my own life, I hope that this chapter can illuminate not just differences and why they exist, but also shed light on some common ground shared between advocates and professionals.

I believe there are many ways in which the interests of advocates and professionals intersect. I am proposing in this chapter that fostering partnerships and collaborations between advocates and professionals can be an effective strategy for improving public attitudes and behaviours toward PWS. This chapter includes: (1) an explanation of differences between advocates and professionals that may result in tension; (2) descriptions of how the interests of advocates and professionals can overlap; (3) a description of evidence-based strategies for reducing public stigma and increasing positive attitudes toward PWS; and (4) ideas for future collaborations between advocates and professionals to improve public attitudes toward stuttering. I hope that both advocates and professionals in the area of stuttering reading this chapter will consider how their capacity to help PWS can be supported by these advocate–professional collaborations.

I also want to inform you of my own background and experiences and how they inform my views. I am a researcher in the area of stuttering who has spent several years investigating stigma experienced by PWS and ways to reduce it. I am a clinical speech-language pathologist who has assessed and treated PWS of various ages. I previously developed and led a self-help/support group for adults who stutter. Importantly, I am a person who stutters and have experience coping with stuttering and its effects. Throughout this chapter I will be providing different perspectives that my own life experiences have given me. In discussing the topic of partnerships between advocates and professionals, I will be referring to certain evidence that has informed my views, my own scientific research to back up some of my claims, and my own personal views based on my experiences throughout life, including those as a client of speech therapy and a clinician who provides services to PWS.

Differences in addressing stigma between advocates and professionals

I believe that a variety of professionals can and should serve as advocates for PWS; however, for the sake of discussion, in this chapter I will be referring to 'professionals' as clinically certified speech-language pathologists or researchers in the field of communication sciences and disorders, and 'advocates' as individuals focused on disability rights for PWS who are not professional speech-language pathologists or researchers in that field. There are several differences between these groups that can explain tensions that exist. These differences include: (a) agendas and goals; (b) how goals are achieved; (c) defining of successful outcomes; and (d) theoretical frameworks, or models of disability that are emphasized.

Patrick Corrigan, a researcher focusing on the stigma of mental illness, wrote an article in 2016 for the journal *World Psychiatry* in which he described some tensions that can occur between advocates and professionals, and I will be referring to his ideas frequently in this chapter. At a basic level, tensions can exist because some advocates have felt disenfranchised by professionals or had negative experiences with them. Many consumer-based, grassroots advocacy groups may have been created because of dissatisfaction with professional services. In addition, advocates are facing difficult situations on a daily basis related to public stigma and social injustices. These advocates may feel like they need to act immediately to correct these injustices, and that they do not have the luxury to seek professional advice regarding best practices for improving public attitudes. They might also feel they cannot wait until research has been published in this area before acting to try to improve social conditions.

The two groups may have different agendas and goals. As Corrigan described in a 2015 article published in the journal *Psychiatric Services*, and again in a 2016 article in the *British Journal of Psychiatry*, professionals may be involved more in a *services agenda* to reduce stigma, whereas advocates might be focused on more of a *rights agenda*. Although they can certainly overlap, discussing them in different categories will help with this discussion and help you to understand why tensions can exist.

A services agenda

A services agenda seeks to increase care seeking of PWS by removing stigma. For example, a professional who writes a newspaper article in a local newspaper to educate the public about stuttering and its treatment options is an example of a services approach. The goal of that approach is to demystify stuttering and normalize it as a treatable medical condition just like any other, so that individuals who stutter and their families can better recognize the condition and be fully educated about their options for managing it. If misunderstandings exist among the public (e.g., mistaken beliefs that stuttering is a psychological problem, or simply a behaviour that one could stop if desired), these can lead to stigma about stuttering and PWS might be less willing to come forward and seek help because of embarrassment or shame.

Public service campaigns focused on education and impression management are very often the vehicle for this approach. For example, contrasting myths with facts about stuttering (e.g., discussing research on physical causes) that highlight the idea that PWS are normal and fundamentally no different from anyone else, are often utilized. In my own research I have seen the benefits of public education in stuttering through improved public attitudes. Many people simply do not understand stuttering or what causes it. They often mistake it for an intellectual disability or a psychological problem.

Professionals who push the services agenda are individuals who are confident that treatment does help, and they may have had their own positive therapy experiences. I have had my share of therapy experiences that were helpful, although some were not. Also, some of the therapy experiences that seemed unhelpful at the time became helpful to me later in life. Because I have seen the positive potential of stuttering therapy as both a client and clinician, I believe that treatment can have a positive impact on the lives of PWS.

Professionals normally use interactive models of disability such as the environmental model, or functional model, which define disability as an interaction between the individual and their environment. The biopsychosocial model described by the World Health Organization is an example of an interactive model that accounts for both personal and environmental factors. It is also used by the American Speech-Language-Hearing Association. The services agenda promotes the idea that there are strategies that can help PWS alter their speech production to become less tense and effortful, and help improve thoughts and feelings about themselves and their communication. If PWS feel stigmatized they may not seek this help, or stay involved in therapy. The services agenda is normally supported by professional service providers and their professional organizations. Success, according to this agenda, would be defined as more PWS seeking services, becoming more engaged in them, and therefore improving their quality of life and communicative participation.

A rights agenda

In contrast to the services approach often utilized by professionals, advocates might focus more on a rights agenda, which intends to eliminate discrimination and social injustice felt by PWS and replace them with affirming and supportive attitudes. This approach focuses on the right of PWS to have opportunities in life given reasonable accommodations. An example could be a presentation to the public, or specific target audience of employers or educators, in which a panel of PWS discuss barriers they have faced in specific settings and provide recommendations for how these barriers could be removed.

I have presented in panels of individuals with disabilities for Disability Awareness Month in the United States to discuss stuttering with members of the public and share my perspective on the condition and how certain listener reactions can be harmful. I have also provided recommendations for how listeners should react. Rather than focus on normalcy, the rights agenda emphasizes and celebrates the differences of PWS by promoting acceptance and pride of stuttering and being a PWS. In this agenda, solidarity is often emphasized, which means standing with others who are in the minority. A sense of pride can come from feelings of overcoming challenges associated with stuttering (e.g., demonstrating resilience and fighting stigma), or simply the realization that stuttering is an aspect of people that has helped shape their lives and who they have become.

The realization can also be gained that there may be several positive outcomes which people have experienced in their life as a result of their stuttering. This acceptance can also engender feelings of authenticity and the understanding that disability can be a source of self-actualization. In my own life I have realized that stuttering has been a major factor in shaping me into the person that I am today and that many of the most important relationships I have developed in my life were a result of stuttering. In that way, I believe stuttering can be perceived as a gift and a source of pride. Although I must say that it has been a long and ongoing process to come to some of these realizations, and there are certainly times in my daily life when I view stuttering as an annoyance or hindrance rather than a gift.

The rights agenda is normally pushed by individuals who have had experiences with prejudice or discrimination, either directly or through observing the experiences of others, and it is often more grassroots in nature. These grassroots advocacy campaigns include PWS who challenge social barriers locally. These individuals might focus more on the social model of disability (also called the minority model, or sociopolitical model) which defines disability as socially constructed, and views individuals with disabilities as belonging to a minority group that is denied its full civil rights. This model is newer than the others previously mentioned and is also radically different from them.

Success, according to the rights agenda, would mean that PWS are being discriminated against less and are instead receiving accommodations that help them succeed. Some advocates using this model might resist medical categorizations and diagnoses of their condition because they believe this may intensify stigma. They may also minimize reliance on professionals or academics who are so-called 'experts'. Instead of turning to experts, these advocates seek self-determination and the freedom to define for themselves what stuttering means and how it affects their lives.

In summary, there are a variety of ways in which advocates and professionals differ regarding their handling of stigma experienced by PWS. The differences reflect the various roles, training, and backgrounds of these individuals. As I mentioned previously, these agendas are not mutually exclusive and ideally there would be plenty of overlap between them. For example, professionals can and certainly should act as advocates. I suppose I am an example of this given that I act as both a professional who believes in the positive potential of therapy and an advocate who brings societal discrimination and prejudice to public awareness.

Although there is the possibility of overlap, from my own experience I have seen energetic debate and disagreement about how to look at stuttering between individuals who I would categorize as adhering more to either the 'services agenda' or the 'rights agenda'. Despite these differences, which can create tension and debate, there are many ways in which the services agenda and the rights agenda can converge to improve public attitudes about stuttering, as is described in more detail in the next section.

Goals of advocates and professionals can complement each other

Relationships between advocacy and clinical work

Depending on the situation, there can be cases in daily life in which either professionals' service agenda or advocates' rights agenda might be more useful for reaching certain goals. For example, normalcy messages may be more effective in reducing stigma so that treatment can be sought. An example of how the services agenda can complement the rights agenda comes from my own professional experience. I once wrote an educational article about stuttering for a local newspaper in a rural town in the United States. The article discussed how to identify stuttering, risk factors for persistence, and recommendations for assessment and treatment from a certified speech-language pathologist. After the article was published, a close colleague of mine in the school system of that town told me that she started receiving more requests for evaluations and treatment of students who stutter.

In one case in particular, a mother stated that her teenage son had been struggling with stuttering since he was very young, but the family never talked about it. They had once heard early in this child's life that nothing could be done about stuttering. For over fifteen years, the child was very limited in his communication socially and in the classroom and rarely, if ever, discussed stuttering with anyone else. I consulted with his therapist and a plan was developed for therapy that included speech modification goals, as well as promoting a sense of empowerment through voluntary stuttering, and advertising and discussing stuttering openly. In a few months this teenager was participating in class, and talking with a classmate he had always been interested in dating but never spoke to due to his fear of stuttering. In fact, not only did he speak to her, but he spoke to her about his stuttering. At the end of his therapy, this client described voluntary stuttering as his favourite therapy strategy, and expressed his desire to become a speech-language pathologist.

Through this example it can be seen that reducing stigma through education in the service model can help PWS feel empowered to become their own advocates and educate others about stuttering. These behaviours that the client developed with the assistance of therapy helped him to become his own advocate and to promote more understanding and acceptance of stuttering at home, school, and his social environments.

The rights agenda and emphasizing solidarity might be particularly relevant for some people with self-stigma related to their stuttering at particularly difficult times in their lives. These individuals might need the support from peers who stutter with whom they can share experiences and learn from. As an example, a former self-help member of a local chapter that I ran for PWS commented that even though he thought therapy was very beneficial, there was an extra ingredient in self-help that he found unique and powerful. The idea of simply being able to talk to other PWS was incredibly empowering and comforting to him. He reported that in our group meetings, he could be himself and that it was the only time in his life in which he felt accepted completely as he was, not needing to "do anything" for anyone else.

Another acquaintance of mine commented that attending the annual convention of the National Stuttering Association and seeing other individuals who stutter, who were also successful and pursuing their goals, was the single biggest catalyst for his ability to feel more empowered himself regarding his employment options. Importantly, many speech-language pathologists that I know who are knowledgeable in stuttering educate clients about self-help opportunities, such as local self-help meetings, or larger national conventions for PWS. Many attendees at self-help conventions aimed at empowering PWS are made aware of these opportunities by professionals in the field of speech-language pathology.

Professionals can also empower clients by using their knowledge of the field and sharing resources likes books, videos, and podcasts, from organizations like the Stuttering Foundation, National Stuttering Association, Friends, or StutterTalk, which seek to discuss stuttering openly and help connect PWS. These examples demonstrate that there is overlap in the services provided by professionals and the rights agenda of advocates. I believe the examples just mentioned illustrate the fact that even though specific agendas or approaches may be more or less effective with certain people at different points in time, they both have an important role and can overlap in their ultimate goals of improving communicative participation and quality of life for individuals who stutter.

Relationships between advocacy and research

In addition to overlap and partnerships between advocates and clinical speech-language pathologists, the intersection of advocacy and research is critical to address. Advocates face social injustices on a daily basis, and they often act quickly to prevent these acts from occurring. These intentions can sometimes backfire, however, because not all attempts to improve public attitudes are successful. In fact, several research studies have documented that certain anti-stigma strategies (e.g., showing people documentaries about stuttering, or coursework on stuttering) have little to no effect on attitudes about stuttering, and some even intensify negative attitudes. If you are interested in reading more about these studies, I recommend reading a book edited by Ken St. Louis in 2015, called *Stuttering Meets Stereotype, Stigma, and Discrimination: An Overview of Attitude Research*.

Because of the possibility of unintended consequences that can make situations worse rather than better, it is critical that advocates utilize validated strategies established by research as being effective in reaching those desired goals. If professional organizations or local grassroots advocacy groups are spending limited time and resources to reduce public stigma about stuttering, they should choose evidence-based strategies from scientific studies. In the next section, I will briefly describe some research findings that my students and I documented as being important for reducing public stigma for PWS.

Different ways to challenge public stigma related to stuttering

Recent research that I have conducted with my students at Montclair State University focused on gaining evidence for specific types of anti-stigma approaches for stuttering that can be used with members of the public. In 2016, a study that I conducted along with my graduate student assistants was published in the *Journal of Fluency Disorders*. The study compared the effects of three anti-stigma strategies – protest, education, and contact – on thoughts, emotions, and anticipated behaviour toward PWS. The strategies of protest, education, and contact were described by Corrigan and Kosyluk in a 2013 article in the journal *Basic and Applied Social Psychology* in the context of mental illness stigma. In our experiment we applied these strategies to stuttering.

Protest seeks to condemn and rebuke negative stereotypes and actions that are observed in the public. For example, if someone in the media mocks stuttering, a press release can be made on behalf of PWS that criticizes that behaviour (e.g., "It is never okay to make fun of stuttering. Shame on you for perpetuating these negative views!"). Protest is normally expressed in a way that conveys moral indignation or righteous anger at the offenders.

Education uses a more neutral tone and highlights common myths about stuttering. These myths are then paired with facts or current scientific evidence in the area of stuttering (e.g., "MYTH: stuttering is psychological, and is caused by tension or nervousness. FACT: stuttering is a neurodevelopmental condition with a strong genetic component").

Contact involves the public hearing a personal story from an individual with lived experience with the condition. For example, a PWS might share a personal story, highlighting both the challenges faced as well as perseverance in the face of obstacles. Individuals utilizing a contact approach would also describe success they have had in life, as well as specific goal statements that they want the audience to take away from the encounter (e.g., telling the listeners how to act or respond when talking with PWS).

Research summary on anti-stigma approaches for stuttering

In our study, we randomly assigned 212 adults in the United States to watch one of four possible 5-minute videos related to anti-stigma strategies for stuttering: protest, education, contact, or a control group which received no information about stuttering. Participants completed a series of questions before, immediately after, and one week after watching one of these four videos. Results showed that all three anti-stigma approaches led to significantly reduced negative stereotypes, negative emotional reactions, and discriminatory intentions compared to the control condition immediately after watching the video. Stereotypes were significantly reduced for those individuals in the education and protest groups, compared to the control group, one week after they watched the video. However, the contact group was the only group that reported significantly higher ratings of affirming attitudes toward PWS compared to the control group, after watching the video and one week later. Therefore, it seems that these different strategies can be used to achieve different aims.

Although education and protest seem very effective for reducing negative attitudes, contact might be most useful for increasing affirming attitudes.

Participants in the contact, education, and protest conditions all reported an increased understanding of stuttering that was significantly greater than the control group. In addition, participants reported enjoying watching the videos. Participants in the education and contact groups self-reported significantly more positive attitude change about stuttering as a result of watching the video, compared with the control group. The protest group was not significantly different from the control group regarding self-reported positive attitude change. Additionally, every single participant in the contact group reported a better understanding of stuttering and reported that they enjoyed the video, and this was not the case for education and protest. Importantly, no participants in either contact, education, or protest conditions reported a less positive attitude about PWS after the experiment.

Therefore, to summarize the findings of our study it seems that although education, contact, and protest can be beneficial in different ways, personal contact might be particularly useful to improve understanding of stuttering and increase positive attitudes. Other research studies have documented the beneficial effects of education and personal contact for improving positive attitudes and reducing negative attitudes about PWS. For more detail on these studies, I recommend reading St. Louis's 2015 book on the subject.

In 2017, my students and I published a follow-up study in the journal *Speech, Language and Hearing* that identified the key elements of the protest, education, and contact programmes mentioned previously. Participants who watched these videos explained that there were several features of protest and education that improved their attitudes, including dispelling myths and replacing them with facts about stuttering; highlighting examples of successful individuals who stutter who also have high speech demand jobs; and emphasizing that, despite differences in speech, PWS are just like anyone else. Elements of the contact condition that improved attitudes included the presenter being a PWS with lived experience, the content including stories of challenges faced as well as the recovery process, and the presenter making a clear request for affirming behaviours toward PWS (e.g., stating how we would like to be treated, or how to interact with PWS).

I believe these findings will help advocates develop anti-stigma campaigns that include validated content to achieve their aims. In addition, we hope that a fidelity measure can be generated from these results which would help to identify the strengths of various anti-stigma programmes for stuttering.

Interestingly, I have felt the impact of these strategies in my own life as well. From my research I have seen evidence to support the notion that being open about stuttering and sharing experiences with others increases positive attitudes. In my personal life I often feel a sense of empowerment when I talk openly about my stuttering to other people. In my view, being open about stuttering and talking about it with the public seems to serve two purposes: improving public attitudes of the individuals in my environment and increasing my own personal sense of empowerment.

Future collaborations between advocates and professionals

Professionals (speech-language pathologists) will continue to emphasize service delivery to help empower PWS and provide them with options about how to best manage stuttering. These professionals can also refer clients to various self-help and support groups and conferences in order for them to develop personal relationships with other PWS, and stand in solidarity with these individuals. Advocacy and self-help/support group networks focusing on the rights agenda often rely on professionals for making PWS aware that these options exist and could be pursued. It should be reiterated that both therapy for stuttering from a professional and seeking support from other PWS are not mutually exclusive. However, it seems that each one contains unique aspects that cannot be obtained from the other. Therefore, in my judgement they may both be incredibly valuable for different people depending on their needs at different points in their lives, and certainly many PWS are involved in these activities concurrently.

Regarding research, advocates should seek out current evidence for guidance on selecting and implementing anti-stigma strategies to achieve their goals. Advocates' use of research findings to inform their advocacy campaigns is critical for improving public attitudes. It is important moving forward that there is a relationship between professionals and advocates so that each group can learn from the other, and we can together maximize our ability to improve public attitudes and behaviours toward PWS.

From the research I have conducted, and the research of my colleagues, I can see evidence that both a services agenda (focused on education about stuttering), and a rights agenda (focused on personal contact and highlighting social injustices) can be beneficial in improving public attitudes. Therefore, partnerships between individuals focused on the services agenda and those focused on the rights agenda could result in maximally effective anti-stigma campaigns.

Certainly, tensions will continue to exist between these two agendas and it is possible that there are unintended consequences of a services agenda that would be directly in conflict with the rights agenda. For example, could PWS interpret professionals' recommendations for therapy as invalidating a part of who they are? Would PWS interpret stuttering as their individual problem and ignore the problems in society? Clearly, future research needs to continue investigating similarities and differences between these types of approaches and their effects on attitudes, and document any of their unintended negative consequences. This is especially true given the fact that these different approaches will likely be competing for limited funding, and choices must be made about the best ways to improve public attitudes about stuttering.

Despite these conflicts, I believe it is beneficial to focus on the common ground shared between these approaches and maintain an optimistic perspective about collaboration going forward. Professionals must realize that they can contribute to changing social conditions for PWS. As mentioned earlier, the terms 'advocate' and 'professional' represent a false dichotomy because individuals can be both of these things. Speech-language pathologists and researchers should take action to reduce stigma through advocacy efforts at institutional and political levels. Although assessment and treatment of PWS by professionals can certainly help to create societal changes, professionals' roles should extend beyond this. For example, advocating for public policies to support PWS, modifying environmental barriers for increased participation of PWS, and alerting the public to stereotypes, prejudice, and discrimination against PWS are particularly important. Professionals can work on these goals individually or in collaboration with local, state, or national organizations.

The importance of empowering people who stutter

Professionals should also consider that although they may possess clinical expertise and knowledge regarding service delivery for PWS, this does not mean that they alone should take the primary role for changing social conditions for PWS. As Patrick Corrigan described in his work on mental illness stigma, it is critical for professionals to realize that people with lived experience are best situated to drive the effort for changing how our society thinks about stuttering. Professionals bring resources and credibility to the table which can be very important for public attitude change, and they can play a supportive role to improve social conditions. However, PWS themselves are best positioned to promote the agenda of their community in terms of actions and policies that affect their lives.

If stigma represents an imbalance of power, strong leadership from PWS represents a shift in power to the minority group. If professionals try to be the sole driving force of these social efforts, it may unintentionally disempower PWS. Therefore, the adage "Nothing about us without us" is a critical message to remember as it represents the important notion that policies and actions related to a group should be considered with full participation of that group. Often, in the area of stuttering, service providers (speech-language pathologists) have their own personal history as a PWS. These professionals can be particularly influential in their ability to share their own experiences as service recipients and providers, and can promote the stigma change agenda through a variety of professional outlets such as writings or presentations. For example, some of my colleagues and I speak at national and international professionals' conferences and describe our perspectives as PWS and advocates who are also speech-language pathologists. I have seen firsthand that these types of presentations are of interest to many people, and the response is overwhelmingly positive.

A personal reflection and conclusion

One final point that I want to emphasize is that interpersonal contact with PWS seems to be one of the most effective ways for improving public attitudes about stuttering according to the evidence. It is important to state at the end of this chapter that this personal contact, which my own research and personal experience has shown to be effective, is dependent upon PWS acknowledging their stuttering, disclosing it, and talking about it openly with other people in their communities. Despite this knowledge, I sometimes experience periods of speech fluency that seem to disassociate me from the identity of a person who stutters. I often enjoy the times in which fluent speech comes easily in my everyday life. I know many other PWS who feel the same.

However, a negative consequence of these periods of fluency for me is that it becomes tempting to habitually avoid identifying as a person who stutters in everyday interactions. This can be problematic because if stuttering continues to be invisible, the rights agenda cannot be advanced. Instead of being tempted to hide or minimize stuttering, both professionals and advocates who stutter need to realize that they can serve as incredibly powerful change agents to reduce stigma. Although there are certainly risks to being open about stuttering (e.g., experiencing public stigma), it will be helpful to remind ourselves that we have the power to challenge public stigma by disclosing our stuttering, discussing it openly, and educating others to create a more understanding society. It is my hope that this chapter provides both advocates and professionals some useful ideas for improving societal attitudes about stuttering, and how they might work cooperatively to achieve this important goal.

References

Boyle, M.P., Dioguardi, L., & Pate, J.E. (2016). A comparison of three strategies for reducing the public stigma associated with stuttering. *Journal of Fluency Disorders, 50*, 44-58.

Boyle, M.P., Dioguardi, L., & Pate, J.E. (2017). Key elements in contact, education, and protest based anti-stigma programs for stuttering. *Speech, Language and Hearing, 20*, 232-240.

Corrigan, P.W. (2015). Challenging the stigma of mental illness: Different agendas, different goals. *Psychiatric Services, 66*, 1347-1349.

Corrigan, P.W. (2016). Lessons learned from unintended consequences about erasing the stigma of mental illness. *World Psychiatry, 15*, 67-73.

Corrigan, P.W. (2016). Resolving mental illness stigma: Should we seek normalcy or solidarity? *The British Journal of Psychiatry, 208*, 314-315.

Corrigan, P.W. & Kosyluk, K.A. (2013). Erasing the stigma: Where science meets advocacy. *Basic and Applied Social Psychology, 35*, 131–140.

St. Louis, K.O. (Ed.), (2015). *Stuttering Meets Stereotype, Stigma, and Discrimination: An Overview of Attitude Research.* Morgantown, WV: West Virginia University Press.

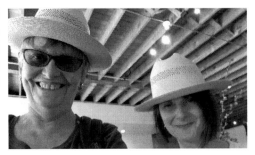

Carolyn Cheasman (left) and Rachel Everard (right) trying on stetsons in Texas after running an Acceptance and Commitment Therapy workshop for people who stammer.

A tale of two therapists

Rachel Everard and Carolyn Cheasman

We are two speech and language therapists who both stammer and work at City Lit, a national UK centre in adult stammering therapy. In this chapter, we re-evaluate our personal experiences of stammering and our professional practice through the social model of disability lens, reflecting on possible sources of public and self-stigma and exploring how our beliefs about stammering influence our work. What follows are personal descriptions of how we have consciously and subconsciously been influenced by the way stammering has been perceived over the course of our lifetimes and what that has meant to us as people who stammer and in our work as speech and language therapists.

Rachel's story

Dear Reader,

I would like to take you on a journey, a very personal one, where I draw upon my experience as a person who stammers and a speech and language therapist (SLT) to explore my engagement with the social model of disability and stammering. I must confess that when I normally attempt to write something, I am filled with apprehension as writing does not come easily to me. However, this feels different because of the personal nature of what I'm going to write and I am wondering who you, as a reader, might be. Perhaps you're someone who stammers, or a speech and language therapist, or someone who for personal or professional reasons is interested in stammering. Whoever you might be, I hope you will be able to take something away from what you're about to read.

Another reason why this experience of writing feels positively liberating is because I've been given strict instructions **not** to make it into an academic text, with the inclusion of references to back up the points I want to make. It is a luxury to write from my own direct and personal experience.

So, let's get to the matter in hand – how do I engage with the social model of disability in the context of stammering? I'll put my cards on the table straightaway and admit I have varied and conflicting emotions regarding the social model of disability and how it applies to my own stammering and to my work with people who stammer.

This conflict dates back to my own experiences of stammering as a young child. I started stammering as soon as I started speaking, at the age of 3, in the 1960s, and as far as I can remember stammering was never openly discussed in our household. I think this was partly due to the fact that not much of emotional content was ever discussed – remember this was a long time ago in middle-class England where the mantra 'keep a stiff upper lip' was part of my cultural upbringing.

When considering my family's response to stammering, it is also important to take into account that my mother has a stammer. From what she has subsequently told me, she stammered much more as a young child and was teased about her stammering by her siblings and cousins. So she grew up with the strong external message that stammering is something to be ridiculed and as a result quickly learned to hide it as well as she could. Then at a young age she met, fell in love with, and married my father, starting life with him far away in America. She has often described marrying my father as a turning-point in her life when she stopped stammering (or when it became much less of an issue). Having gone through those difficult childhood experiences, it must have been very hard for my mother to have had a child of her own who stammers, and I think I quickly picked up that stammering was something to be hidden and never discussed. This reluctance to talk about stammering within the family most likely was also encouraged at the time, in the hope that it would by itself naturally disappear.

I had speech therapy around the age of 11; it was just me and a therapist who taught me syllable-timed speech. No-one else in my family was involved and we never discussed my stammering or the therapy I was receiving. I remember enjoying the sessions with the therapist, who was kind and understanding, and with her I could speak freely and easily. Not surprisingly I never made use of the syllable-timed speech she taught me – it sounded far too weird to me as a self-conscious child. I just learnt to hide the stammering ever more deeply and I think it was assumed by my family and teachers, in a well-meaning way, that I was 'cured', that speech therapy had helped me overcome stammering. They could not have been more wrong – it was just driven underground.

From my story so far, you will probably understand that I came to think about stammering as something that was shameful, just as my mother had done. So, from a social model perspective, I internalized many of the unspoken negative beliefs about stammering and came to see it as an unacceptable part of me, which I became successful in hiding. The way I was encouraged to manage my stammering was from a medical model perspective – I was the person with the problem, so I was the one who needed to deal with it and learn to speak like everyone else by learning a fluency technique, which in my case was syllable-timed speech.

I would describe the way I stammer now as interiorized or covert, where I have a fair amount of natural fluency, a tendency to avoid stammering through a variety of strategies, and in the past strong negative feelings around stammering which have lessened over the years through therapy. Would it be fair to say that I interiorized my stammering because of the stigma I experienced as a child? It seems to be a plausible explanation as to why I chose to hide my stammer: if a child openly stammers and then picks up, over time, via external messages from family, peers, teachers and therapists that stammering behaviours are undesirable, a natural response would be to develop feelings of shame, fear, embarrassment and frustration and a whole raft of increasingly sophisticated avoidance strategies. More on this later.

The turning point came for me when, in my 20s, I attended group therapy at City Lit, the specialist centre in adult stammering therapy where I now work. Up to that point, I had gone to enormous lengths to hide my stammering, even turning down a job as I thought I would be unable to say the company's name when answering the phone. It was an extraordinary and positive experience to be with other people who stammer, for stammering to be talked about openly, and to feel accepted, stammer and all. From a social model perspective, I no longer felt different but part of a community. I was able to challenge some of the negative beliefs about stammering I had held for so long, but it was a slow process. What helped was joining other communities of people who stammer, and I became active in the British Stammering Association (BSA) for a number of years. Therapy enabled me to develop a more robust identity of myself as a PWS and from this position I was better equipped to make choices about what I wanted to do with my life. I decided to train as a speech and language therapist.

During my time as a trustee of the BSA, I remember a debate about the BSA vision. Two alternatives were proposed – a world without stammering and a world that understands stammering. Looking back at this from a disability model perspective, I can see the former takes a medical model stance, i.e., stammering is unwanted, therefore let's get rid of it, whereas the latter is about embracing difference, more in line with the social model. At the time I was in favour of a world without stammering and argued forcefully that if people who stammer had the choice, they would prefer not to stammer at all. It is interesting for me to reflect how far I have changed my thinking on this subject. If I were involved in this debate again, I would definitely support the vision that was ultimately and very wisely chosen: a world that understands stammering.

My shift towards the social model has been gradual and still continues. I feel drawn to it because I believe it explains, to a large extent, the amount of shame and fear people who stammer often experience. Why should taking longer to say something give rise to so many negative thoughts and feelings? This level of discomfort with stammering is more easily understood when stammering is put in a social context – people who stammer fear the negative judgement of others because their speech sounds different. And I believe that it is partly because of the fear of negative judgement that a lot of struggle behaviour develops and many of the avoidance behaviours emerge.

Having said that, I do not think the stigma experienced by people who stammer can wholly explain struggle and avoidance behaviour. For me personally, the physical act of stammering is itself uncomfortable, regardless of how others may be judging my speech, and part of the struggle and avoidance behaviour is a natural consequence of trying to get away from that uncomfortable feeling.

It is tantalising to contemplate the idea that if there was no stigma associated with stammering, would people stammer less? If a child started to stammer and was totally accepted for who they were and how they spoke, would they continue to stammer? Or would they continue to stammer without any struggle or avoidance? From my own experience as someone who stammers and from working with many people who stammer, I strongly believe that it is the repeated struggle not to stammer that perpetuates and prolongs the physical moments of stammering and that it is the avoidance of stammering that reinforces the fear of stammering.

So where does this leave me as a SLT? I believe that a key role of the SLT is educating others about different ways of looking at stammering and opening people's eyes to the fact that the medical model pervades the world of speech and language therapy without us being conscious of its overriding influence. I think it would be fair to say that most parents of children who stammer and most adults who stammer, when first seeking help, assume that therapy will be about fluency.

Some people who stammer go to huge lengths to make themselves more fluent, often by learning a fluency shaping technique which they have to practise every day and which can cost a significant amount of energy, time and, in some cases, money. They do all this because they want to be 'normal speakers', whatever that might mean. This is very much acting from the medical model perspective – I've got something wrong with me, so I need to change this to be like everyone else. This is a choice people who stammer make without possibly being fully aware of alternative ways of viewing stammering. Helping people to make informed choices about whether to have therapy (and if so, what kind) or to have no therapy is what I believe is important.

I also believe for myself that it is possible to operate from a social model standpoint whilst continuing to support people to stammer more easily, i.e., to work on the impairment itself. When I meet someone whose severity of overt stammering is impacting their ability to lead the life they want, I believe work on the stammer itself can be helpful, as long as that is what they want. The challenge, for me, is conveying an attitude of acceptance whilst at the same time supporting someone to develop an easier pattern of speech.

I have heard on more than one occasion the view that some levels of stammering are acceptable whereas some levels of stammering are not. So, if someone stammers once in a while and it is perceived (and it is interesting to consider who is making this judgement – the listener or the speaker?) that the stammering does not affect the person's ability to get their message across, then that's OK. But if someone stammers on every word to the extent that it is difficult without a lot of effort on the part of the listener to understand the message, then that is not acceptable. Although I have understanding for the latter position and have, I must admit, on a number of occasions caught myself thinking when listening to someone with a very severe overt stammer, "Oh, they could really do with some speech work", I understand that from a social model perspective all levels of types and stammering need to be equally accepted.

I now work from the premise that it is the client's view that is paramount in all of this, but here we encounter a dilemma. Take, for example, the young man who came to see me: a bright articulate student who has stammered since childhood, who views his stammering as 'crippling', and who has experienced mental health difficulties because of it. He is an extremely long way from accepting his stammering; in fact, all he wants to do is get rid of it as fast as he can. His choice would be to learn a fluency technique, but if I were to go along with this, would I not be colluding with his strongly-felt belief that stammering is bad and fluency is good? At the same time, if I were to encourage him to accept his stammering in the early stages of therapy, I might alienate him. It takes a skilful therapist to provide the right amount of support and education so that the person who stammers feels understood and sees a way forward.

One argument, convincing in my view, put forward by disability activists is that stammering could be seen as a variation of speech, in the same way we all speak with different accents. Just as it is acceptable to have a different accent, so it is acceptable to speak with different levels of fluency. However, one important aspect of stammering complicates the situation: its variability. If you're a person who stammers, you'll know only too well that sometimes you'll stammer a lot, sometimes a little and sometimes not at all. To the outsider this begs the question: "Well, if you can speak fluently some of the time, why can't you speak fluently all of the time?" For the person who stammers it can be deeply frustrating to speak easily some of the time but not all of the time. It's harder to accept something that fluctuates from moment to moment; it's easier to accept something that's always there.

So, there we are, my thoughts around stammering and the social model of disability. Like stammering, they are also in a state of flux. For me the key lies in skilfully educating others about different ways of considering stammering and how these might impact on stammering therapy, so that people who stammer can make an informed choice as to what they wish to gain from therapy, or if they need therapy at all.

Carolyn's story

My earliest memory of stammering is when I was 9. I was standing up at the front of the church congregation and suddenly felt I could not get a word out. I immediately and instinctively resorted to avoidance to cope – I am not sure I even knew what 'it' was then – did I have a name for it? I do know it went completely underground from that moment on.

I now recognize I had developed what we call interiorized or covert stammering. From the outside I did not stammer at all and, as I had very high levels of fluency, I found I could keep it hidden by changing words and staying quiet in some situations. I do not remember encountering negative attitudes to stammering because no one knew, so where did my instinctive desire to hide it come from? Right from the beginning, I had found it inherently uncomfortable to feel out of control of my behaviour and I did not like that feeling. There seemed to be some shame attached to doing this thing and, I guess, to feeling different. I was growing up in a British middle-class 1950s/1960s culture that probably valued conformity and not being different. I had sat next to a boy at school who stammered frequently and with struggle. Had I picked up messages about him and found it uncomfortable to hear him speak?

It is interesting that despite no memory of direct messages about my stammering, I immediately decided to hide it. Arriving at secondary school and being faced with having to read out loud in class, I told my parents about my stammering and said I would like to be excused from reading. It must have been very hard for them to understand what was going on because they had never heard me stammer, but they were aware of my very high levels of anxiety. I was duly excused from oral reading.

Looking back as an experienced SLT, I can look at this as a generalized collusion to help me avoid stammering. As such, this was probably an unhelpful strategy in the long run. Could this be seen within social model thinking as collusion with societal mores to maintain 'normality'? It has only recently been pointed out to me that another, and very different, view from a social model stance is that reasonable adjustments were made to help me cope with a speech impairment. However, there's another interesting layer. Could reasonable adjustments such as this, which would presumably be supported by social model thinking, also be seen to be colluding with the idea that it's best for stammering not to be heard? It's complicated. Whatever, I think that the undergrounding of my stammering was ultimately unhelpful and was part of what led me to make particular life choices. Ultimately, stammering and my feelings about it probably influenced my choice of degree. I might have liked to have done English, but the oral reading requirements led me down the science route.

Like Rachel, I was fortunate to find City Lit later on in my life and was able to start to develop a more useful understanding of my stammering and how to respond to it. Even then, I was exposed to what might be seen as a rather contradictory mix of approaches. Initially, I was encouraged to reduce avoidance behaviours and to start to 'come out' alongside being taught some block modification. At the same time, I was introduced to syllable-timed speech and then, it being the mid 1970s, slow or prolonged speech hit the UK and I learned this in an attempt to not stammer. Of course, I tried my hardest to use this technique to the best of my ability because I was still very much not wanting to stammer.

I was then fortunate to work with an enlightened City Lit therapist who knew that for me the key thing would be for me to let myself stammer and to gradually start to change my response to this. As I started to let myself stammer more overtly I encountered a variety of responses. I still had very high levels of fluency and only occasionally stammered, so the predominant response was one of surprise. When I disclosed that I stammered people would tend to say things like, "Oh, we all do that when we are anxious", sometimes people smiled when I stammered, sometimes they looked away, but I think by and large I did not encounter too much judgement. Much of it was in my own mind. Going to City Lit did change my life and I went on to train as a speech and language therapist and went back to work there in 1979.

As a SLT, I embrace some social model principles and I struggle with others. City Lit stammering therapy has changed and evolved over the years: from my time as a client, when avoidance reduction, block modification and syllable-timed speech were taught; through the relatively short phase of only offering slowed speech courses; to a phase when separate speak-more-fluently and stammer-more-fluently programmes were offered. By the mid-1980s, the approach became a pure stammer-more-fluently one with increasing emphasis being placed on openness and acceptance combined with stammering modification work. Cognitive Behavioural Therapy (CBT) strategies were incorporated in the 1990s and mindfulness interventions woven in from 2006. Influenced by the idea that it was possible to integrate speak-more-fluently and stammering-more-fluently strategies, we started to offer integrated courses in the noughties. First, we introduced a programme based on the American Institute for Stuttering approach which at the time taught vocal fold management alongside a whole host of other interventions, and then a programme influenced by the Institute for Stuttering Treatment and Research (ISTAR) approach in Canada. In the past two years, we have nailed our colours to the 'stammer-more-fluently' mast and have dropped all teaching of fluency techniques. It is interesting to reflect on this journey and to see how it to some extent illustrates ongoing controversies as to how best to help adults who stammer. What led us to make the choices we made – what were the key influences?

Up to about 15 years ago, I had not heard of the social model. I was not really aware of the medical model either – I had not started to categorize therapy approaches in this way – but I have always kicked against the idea of 'treatment' and have never used the word 'patient' to describe someone I have worked with. I certainly never regarded myself as a patient when I was participating in therapy. I have a strong and deeply ingrained resistance to teaching people strategies to try to manage stammering through unhelpful attempts to control or suppress as I believe that such strategies ultimately feed the stammering dynamic. I see this as a dynamic whereby physical tension and struggle are perpetuated and even developed through attempts to try as hard as possible not to stammer. As our work evolved in the 1980s towards a more pure stammer-more-fluently approach, it is interesting to reflect on the influences. Whilst stammer-more-fluently approaches are not social model approaches per se, they do work on cultivating greater openness and acceptance of stammering.

As a team, I do not believe we were directly aware of disability activism, but we were collectively and individually definitely influenced by and involved with feminism, the black and gay rights movements, and the anti-apartheid movement. All of these were looking at ways to challenge and fight back against oppression in its various forms. It would be hard to completely separate this from our work context. By the 1990s, I was working with people who were directly exploring social model of disability thinking and for the first time I encountered the term and was involved with the first self-advocacy group for people who stammer that ran in the mid-1990s. This was clearly a course that was directly addressing how social model thinking might be relevant, helpful and liberating for people who stammer. It's been 45 years now since I had therapy myself and 40 years since I started work as an SLT at City Lit. I have described some of the experiences that have influenced me personally and professionally - people who stammer and colleagues have been key here. Learning more about social model thinking continues to be stimulating and challenging – as ever, it is the ongoing questions that make the work so fascinating.

A joint perspective

Right from the start of group therapy, we make it clear that, from our perspective, "it's OK to stammer" and "it's OK not to stammer". In this way, we are hopefully giving clients permission to be whoever they are and immediately challenging a rule they may have internalized from an early age that it is not OK to stammer. Saying it's OK not to stammer can be helpful for people who have more fluency, who might feel they do not have a right to be there if they compare themselves to others in the group who are stammering more obviously. For many years, we have introduced the iceberg analogy as a way to help people share feelings about stammering as part of the covert identification process. More recently, we have encouraged clients to consider the reasons they have developed these often negative feelings. This can lead on to a discussion about the messages society gives us about stammering.

All of our therapy takes place in groups and this is a key way in which people can start to feel part of a wider community of people who stammer and so assist in the process of developing a more robust and positive sense of self as a person who stammers. Group discussions can enable space for counter narratives to start to develop (e.g., what has stammering taught me?).

Our therapy follows a traditional block modification sequence and starts off with an identification phase. We encourage clients to become curious and interested in moments of stammering. Curiosity can help to develop a very different approach to one which might have been rooted in avoidance, fear or denial. This phase gives opportunities to challenge particular uses of language. For example, people who stammer will often describe stammering as 'bad' and fluency as 'good'. We help people to reflect on this very entrenched way of describing their speech and encourage them to use non-judgemental language. So instead of saying "I stammered really badly just then" they might say "I noticed I was stammering with a lot of tension".

Following identification we move into the desensitization phase of therapy, which aims to help clients open up to the experience of stammering through strategies, like gradually reducing avoidance behaviours, voluntary stammering and self-advertising. Again, this work all supports the development of a more open and accepting sense of self as someone who stammers.

The modification phase introduces clients to ways of reducing the physical tension they experience when they stammer. It is not about eradicating stammering nor replacing it with fluent speech. Some people view any attempts to modify speech behaviours as incompatible with a social model approach. We do not take this view and are careful to approach modification work from a 'letting be/allowing' stance rather than attempts to try to control stammering. We are quite explicit with clients about the unhelpfulness of the word 'control' in relation to stammering. As such, modification is not part of a trying-not-to-stammer process, but almost the opposite. Paradoxically, by allowing themselves to stammer, it becomes less of a physical struggle to speak.

We feel it is important to give clients choices in therapy and one of these choices is having options to speak with less physical tension if that is what they want. We do not subscribe to a more extreme social model position which might argue that any attempts to modify speech collude with societal stigma that stammering is unacceptable. However, it is a fine line that we tread, and the language and approach we take when teaching speech modification strategies is crucial.

As mentioned previously, we have developed a course specifically looking at the social model of disability and how it relates to stammering. A full description of this ground-breaking course, written by St John Harris, can be found in Cheasman, Everard and Simpson (2013). Since the course first ran in 2000, we have continued to run it on a regular basis and it is now called 'You have a voice: self-empowerment for people who stammer'. The aim of the course is to introduce people who stammer to the different ways in which stammering is perceived generally and to illustrate how different models of disability (medical, philanthropic and social) have influenced stammering therapy. It offers the opportunity for participants to engage with these ideas, to discuss them with others and to challenge prevalent stereotypical attitudes and images of stammering.

Challenges

There is no doubt that some of the implications of social model thinking are challenging for us as therapists. One has already been referred to: namely, how much focus to place on stammering modification work. As mentioned earlier, we have in the past experimented with integrating stammer-more-fluently with speak-more-fluently approaches, but finally found the inherent contradiction of encouraging openness about stammering alongside teaching a fluency technique too much. Whilst we are clear that fluency shaping does not fit with our philosophy and approach to therapy, we do still believe in the value of teaching clients stammering modification strategies. Some therapists and people who stammer see this as being at odds with a model that is encouraging clients to be out and proud about stammering. We do not. We believe it is entirely possible to work on acceptance and speech modification, if taught in an allowing/non-suppressing manner, whilst wholeheartedly supporting people who stammer to find value in and embrace their identity.

Another challenge relates to work supporting people to modify their attitudes to stammering, specifically their perceptions of how other people view stammering. We incorporate some CBT to help clients develop a more balanced and realistic view of how stammering is perceived as they often hold strong negative beliefs about stammering. For example, clients frequently express thoughts, such as "if I stammer, people will think less of me" or "I will be seen as less competent in the workplace if I stammer". One of the ways clients are encouraged to challenge these views is by participating in a street survey about stammering where they ask the general public about their views on stammering and people who stammer. Most people come back from this feeling that the majority of those they have stopped genuinely do not hold the negative and prejudicial views they may have anticipated. This is often a very liberating moment for clients.

To what extent should we then balance this with discussion about external barriers, stigma and discrimination? Again, we believe it is a fine line, but one that is possible to tread. We are not trying to push a view that 'everything in the garden is rosy' and there is no negativity or judgement. Our aim is to help people see that some of their automatic assumptions about how others will perceive their stammering are not necessarily accurate. This needs to be balanced with other work around self-esteem and developing a stronger positive identity as people who stammer to help them cope with and challenge discrimination when they experience it.

A further challenge is the often deep-rooted desire for fluency expressed by people who stammer approaching us for help. This desire for fluency is understandable given most people we work with have been stammering since early childhood and have grown up with the message that stammering is an undesirable behaviour and something to be overcome. Our role is to help people understand that focusing on fluency alone is not necessarily the answer and that becoming more open to the experience of stammering can lead to easier speech.

Concluding thoughts

What we have shared here are our personal and professional thoughts around the social model of disability and how we are making sense of it in our work. We hope it is clear that this is very much work in progress and we continue to be influenced by our clients, our colleagues and developments in the field of disability activism. As with many other areas of stammering therapy, there are many more questions than answers, such as:

- Does external stigma of stammering impact on the development of stammering in young children?

- When and how best to educate people who stammer about the different models of disability underlying different models of therapy?

- Whilst social model thinking encourages openness about stammering, can reasonable adjustments which flow from it sometimes collude with stammering not being heard?

- If we as therapists fully espouse social model thinking, should we be doing any impairment-based work at all?

- If we're asking people who stammer to become more accepting of their stammering, do we also have a role as speech and language therapists to encourage greater acceptance of stammering amongst society as a whole?

We would welcome further debate around these issues and the many others that arise out of the impact of social model thinking on stammering, stammering therapy and on the stammering community.

Transforming the stuttering iceberg

Nina G

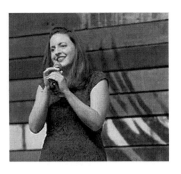

Nina G: Comedian, professional speaker and author of *Stutterer Interrupted: The Comedian Who Almost Didn't Happen*.

When I was in seventh grade, I ran for an office in student body government. When I won the election, whatever excitement I might have felt immediately turned to dread. Getting elected meant having to be sworn into office, which meant saying, "I, Nina G," in front of the whole school – a surefire recipe for public humiliation for a middle schooler who stutters. During rehearsal for the inauguration, the other kids would laugh when I stuttered – I could only imagine what a full auditorium might sound like. There was one slightly older boy named Ahmed, who felt sorry for me; he suggested that I try saying "ninja" and work my way up to "Nina". As you might guess, the random theories of a 12-year-old didn't lead to any breakthroughs. I spent the next week practising my oath of office with my speech therapist, my parents, and my bedroom mirror. When inauguration day came, I stood in front of the school and stuttered. In my seventh grade girl head, I thought my life was over. Who would make fun of me? What school should I transfer to? Would the local paper run a story on what had happened?

The feelings I experienced that day are not uncommon to people who stutter. In fact, there has been a good deal of research on the subject. Joseph Sheehan, clinical psychologist and professor, focused much of his work on the emotional aspects of stuttering. He proposed that what you see and hear in cases of stuttering is just the tip of the iceberg; there are thoughts and feelings occurring under the surface. These internal experiences of stuttering are of much greater importance to the speaker than the surface disfluencies. His theory, appropriately known as Sheehan's iceberg, played a key role in expanding views of stuttering when it was first published in 1970. According to Sheehan, the waterline goes down as the emotions below the surface are confronted and experienced. In theory, the hidden feelings will continue to dissipate until only stuttering remains.

To be clear, Sheehan never claimed that stuttering is caused by emotional issues. His theory was simply that negative emotions can develop as the result of stresses associated with stuttering. In the iceberg model, Sheehan identifies seven different emotions: denial, guilt, fear, shame, isolation, anxiety, and hopelessness. Sheehan believed it was necessary for speech and language pathologists to consider these emotions in order to reveal the full extent of a person's stuttering, which many people conceal through secondary behaviours and avoidance. Examples of my own secondary behaviours include when I start hopping around when I talk on the phone to get out a repetition or time my walking with a word to increase fluency. Problem is, these don't necessarily help over time and can be habit forming. Next thing I know, I am hopping around every time I order a pizza.

The iceberg model is helpful not only to speech and language pathologists, but to other professionals as well (e.g., psychotherapists and social workers), who can help stuttering people process their feelings. My seventh-grade-girl self definitely experienced fear, shame, isolation, anxiety and hopelessness. Back then it would have been helpful to discuss these feelings with a professional; maybe some of the emotional weight that I placed on myself and my speech could have been diffused.

As the stuttering community and the self-help movements gain ground, it is important to consider how Sheehan's model applies to the social model of disability, which takes a social constructivist perspective. Social constructivism considers the interaction of the individual with the environment and how it defines how we think about a particular object or idea at a particular time. For example, if all buildings were ramped or had elevators instead of stairs would a person who uses a wheelchair still be disabled? With physical barriers stripped away, they are able to access everything non-disabled people can. The only potential barriers would be society's poor attitudes and stigmatizing views.

Under the medical model typically used to understand disability and impairments, stuttering is presented in the negative and seen as abnormal. From this viewpoint, stuttering is an aberration that needs to be cured. Although Sheehan's work promoted self-acceptance and community building, he was interested in the consequences of more open and accepting stuttering on the individual, not on society. This focus on the individual has neglected social critique. It has also led to Sheehan's iceberg almost exclusively being used to highlight the negative, personal consequences of stuttering, such as shame, embarrassment, and guilt. I propose that the social model of disability can help us dramatically alter Sheehan's iceberg.

Shifting to the social model of disability, we are able to view stuttering in a more neutral, and even positive, way. In order to show how this shift can effectively happen, we must examine the views of people who stutter, their families, helping professionals, and society at large. Only by understanding the systemic issues can we address what is beneath the tip of the stuttering iceberg. The stuttering iceberg, as well as stuttering itself, can be examined from multiple perspectives.

If you stutter in the woods and no one is around, did you stutter? A systemic model

The social model of disability understands disability as an active process. People are disabled by an environment that does not accommodate their differences and by the negative attitudes and judgements of others. This definition of disability is consistent with the experience of stuttering. Stuttering by itself does not need to foster the negative thoughts and feelings featured in Sheehan's iceberg. Granted, for those of us who stutter the jaw pain from talking after a long day or the frustration of trying to express ourselves is real. Yet I wonder if this frustration would be so intense if we lived in a society more accepting of our speech? Stuttering attendees of any given conference, camp, or support group for people who stutter find this out very quickly. For me, being in an environment free of interruptions and odd reactions to my stutter, as well as being surrounded by people whose speech mirrors my own, has been the single most transformative event in my life.

I have found it important to examine my own ideas about stuttering and, consequently, how my thoughts and feelings are constructed. In particular, Brofrenbrenner's ecological systems theory has helped me to uncover where my own stigmas related to stuttering come from and where to look for more positive images and philosophies.

Uri Brofrenbrenner was a Russian-born American developmental psychologist (for more information see Hayes, O'Toole, & Halpenny, 2017). He proposed that every person is like a Russian nesting doll: the individual is at the core of the doll, with various systems in their environment acting as the surrounding layers. The smaller inner layers represent systems that interact with the individual more directly; the larger outer layers are systems that interact with the individual less directly. Any system can have significant impact on the individual regardless of its distance from the core.

Brofrenbrenner proposed the following systems for his model, arranged from smallest to largest (i.e., most to least direct interaction with the individual):

Microsystem: where the individual interacts with people directly, e.g., family, teachers, therapists, friends, etc.

Mesosystem: where entities in the microsystem interact or communicate with each other without the individual being present, e.g., parent-teacher conferences, teacher lunchtime conversations, friends talking among themselves.

Exosystem: institutions that impact the individual, e.g., libraries, community religious organizations, police, school districts, etc.

Macrosystems: laws, cultural and religious beliefs, media in all forms, etc.

Chronosystem: accounts for the historical period the individual is living in.

These systems can determine the way people think about stuttering. For example, works of fiction traditionally depict people who stutter in a negative light. In movies and literature, characters who stutter tend to be vengeful or pitiful compared to their fluent counterparts. I had a stuttering friend who was in psychotherapy throughout his mid-20s (microsystem interaction). His therapist told him that once he lost his virginity, his stuttering would likely disappear. One can only assume this ignorant remark came from viewing *One Flew Over the Cuckoo's Nest*, in which the stuttering Billy Bibbit has sex and is temporarily fluent (information from the macrosystem). If our stuttering could be cured this way, I am sure many of us would have made that discovery long ago!

This example points to the impact of the macrosystem. People who stutter are rarely portrayed positively in movies and TV shows. Growing up in the 1980s, most people who stuttered I saw in movies either died, killed someone or killed themselves (and were almost always played by actors who did not stutter). Before movies like *Rocket Science* and *King's Speech* came out, the most positive image of a stutterer I saw was a cartoon pig who didn't wear pants (Porky Pig)! As the story of my friend and his therapist demonstrates, these images inform how both society and people who stutter see stuttering.

As a child, I remember my second grade teacher ignoring me when I volunteered to read a prayer at the Catholic school I attended. From that microsystem interaction, I learned that I wasn't a good enough reader to participate in church and school. The teacher didn't say anything, and I am sure she didn't mean to make an impression, but her meaning was implicit to me. It added to the shame Sheehan refers to, which I learned to associate with my stuttering. In high school, the boy I liked (Sean) had his friend talk to my friend about me liking him (mesosystem interaction). The friend said, "Sean would ask Nina out if she wasn't so weird." Neither of them realized that I was affecting 'weirdness' in order to draw attention away from my speech. As Sheehan would say, I was hiding my stuttering through secondary behaviours.

In recent years there was the case of Kylah Simmons, a young woman who was detained at the Atlanta airport for stuttering when questioned by customs. Even though she told them that she stuttered, they said she was lying. As a result, she missed her flight home. In this example, the airport customs is an exosystem (one with poorly trained staff). After the incident, Ms Simmons responded with grace on social media and worked with the Stuttering Foundation to create a travel card that explains stuttering in situations like the one she encountered. Simmons took her negative experience from the microsystem and used it to create a positive interaction affecting the larger exo and macrosystems. Thanks to her, I carry my card everywhere and never leave home without it.

The negative reactions to stuttering in Brofrenbrenner's systems add to the base of Sheehan's iceberg. Sheehan's iceberg theory historically anticipates negative thoughts and feelings as a result of stuttering. For many in the stuttering community, we know that shame, denial, fear, anxiety, isolation, guilt, and hopelessness don't tell our entire story. Examining the stuttering iceberg is like decoding images in the clouds. Depending how you view it, a shape might look like a dragon or a bunny rabbit. In both cases it's the same cloud; our perspective determines what we see. To get the full picture of stuttering, we need to look beyond the negative thoughts and feelings of Sheehan's iceberg and consider a strength-based interpretation. People who stutter – and the professionals working with us – need to know that stuttering can be a source of power and community when viewed in a positive light. Rethinking Sheehan's model from this perspective, we have an opportunity to destigmatize stuttering and step into our own power as communicators. This power comes from both speaking in our everyday life as well as our impacts on our social systems. Much like Ms Simmons' example, our power as communicators transcends the interpersonal realm.

Rethinking the stuttering iceberg

Whether you are a person who stutters, a parent, a speech pathologist, or even work in the media, it is important to consider how you think about stuttering. Do you see it as something that needs to be fixed in order to attain the highest quality of life? Do you believe that people who stutter are destined to live in isolation and hopelessness? If we rely solely on the popular conception of Sheehan's iceberg, we are led to reductive conclusions and forced to overlook the complexities that make up a stuttering person's life.

I'm rarely seen as the merry sunshine type. Not once have I suggested that the power of positive thinking can take away the discrimination and stigma placed on disabled people. That said, I know Sheehan's theory doesn't fully explain my own experience of stuttering, or that of anyone else I know. It is important for us to look at alternative ways of understanding our stuttering experiences and expand from the traditional theories and attitudes we've become accustomed to. Below is my alternative to Sheehan's iceberg, but I encourage readers to construct their own versions.

Sheehan's model places feelings of denial, fear, shame, anxiety, isolation, guilt, and hopelessness beneath the waterline. If we shift to include a more positive perspective on stuttering, we might also experience acceptance, courage, pride, comfort, community, kindness, and hope. This alternate model can help capture the full breadth of our experiences. Remember that story about

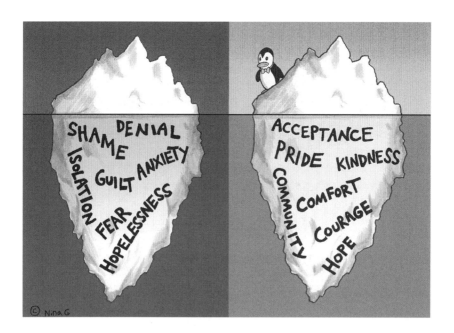

Figure 13.1 Sheehan's iceberg with Nina's alternative iceberg.

me in seventh grade? I left out a few things. After the inauguration ceremony, I got off stage expecting a sea of sadistic children to tease me for the rest of my life. In fact, the only initial response I got was from my classmate Sara. She ran up to me and said, "Nina! Good job!" (I am happy to report that Sara grew up to be a teacher).

Later that day, I was talking with Ahmed (the boy who thought he was helping me with his 'ninja-Nina' theory). We were minding our own business when a third grader came up to us and said, "Hey N-N-N-Nina!" Ahmed told that third grader never to make fun of me again or else he'd publicly embarrass him. It felt good to know someone had my back, and I don't recall being teased much for the rest of that year.

Despite all the positive things that came from me stuttering in front of the school that day, I did not understand it as a positive experience until many years later. I only knew how to focus on the feelings of shame, fear, and anxiety that I experienced. I didn't have any other framework to understand these experiences. If there had been models from my exo and macrosystems that were more empowering, I might have had better tools to transform my internalized stigma. With the alternative iceberg model, I could have viewed my experience back then in terms of courage, comfort, pride, community, kindness, and hope. Eventually, when I was in my 20s, I learned to think about stuttering in positive terms, thanks to the stuttering and Disability communities. these communities taught me how to love myself.

When working with the alternative iceberg model that I have proposed, it's helpful to ask certain questions. These questions are worded from the perspective of a person who stutters, but they can be altered for parents, speech and language pathologists, helping professionals, or anyone else:

- What does stuttering pride mean for me? How will I know when I experience it?

- How will you express pride in your experience of stuttering and the stuttering community? How will you speak with pride and dignity? How will you have the expectations that others will treat you with dignity?

- How do you embody courage? What are some of the things you do to practise courage? (This doesn't have to be giving speeches in front of hundreds of people; it can be posting about stuttering on Facebook, ordering from a drive-thru, or telling a joke at a party.)

- How will you be kind to yourself and others? We sometimes beat ourselves up because of our speech. How can kindness and perhaps forgiveness be part of our experience with stuttering?

- Who do you hope to be with your stuttering (not in spite of it)?

My one fear in writing this chapter is that I don't want people to think there are only two ways to think about stuttering, that you are either in denial or acceptance, shame or pride. Thinking about anything in terms of 'either/or' usually leads to problems. I think there is sometimes a reactionary pressure to view stuttering only in positive terms, probably because we have to compensate for the negative views of society. Still, it's not realistic or even necessary to be one hundred percent positive all the time. Icebergs can hold contradictory feelings. Rather than two separate icebergs, one positive and one negative, perhaps yours holds conflicting elements too? I know people who have said, "I don't see my stuttering as a gift, but I also don't see it as a curse." Ultimately, I hope that stuttering can be more neutral in our lives. We are more than our stutter! We are friends, partners, professionals, and everything else a person can be.

My challenge to the reader, whether or not you stutter, is to examine what your current iceberg looks like and what you want your future iceberg to be. Ideally, I want mine to include pride, but I know there is still shame from my past, like when my second grade teacher didn't pick me to read in front of the school because she assumed I couldn't. When I think of these memories, the negative feelings around stuttering are sometimes highlighted, but then I focus on ways we, as a society, can move forward. Family members and helping professionals can offer support beyond society's narrowly-prescribed response to stuttering. This may include encouraging schools or communities to engage in activities that raise awareness about stuttering. These should go beyond tolerance to embracing the diversity of how people speak. The goal is not about becoming fluent; it is living well with or without fluency.

Reference

Hayes, N., O'Toole, L., & Halpenny, A.M. (2017). *Introducing Bronfenbrenner: A Guide for Practitioners and Students in Early Years Education.* London: Taylor & Francis.

One story at a time: Using a narrative approach in self therapy

Joshua Walker

I'm sitting in the middle row of a big university lecture theatre.

Barry, the university resident musician, is on stage dressed in all black, peering over his synthesizer and Macbook-pro. Off the back of a lengthy tangent – another anecdote about his work with musicians the class has never heard of, Barry chimes, "Next week's topic is 'Spoken Word'. Your job is to find a piece and work on it to perform in class. Any questions?"

Hmmm.

My heart sinks. "I have a question, Barry. What are you doing?! Why are you getting us to do that?! The reason I took a module like 'Exploring the Use of Art in Healthcare' is because I wanted to escape these moments of pressurized speaking. I wanted to mess around on the guitar, sing Wonderwall, and pretend to know how to play the bongos. What happened to contemporary dance week? When are we doing that?"

Of course, rather than voice such strong opinions, I park Barry's task in the avoidance wing of my brain. In fact, I bury it so deep into the recesses of my mind that when next week comes about, I have absolutely no idea what I'm going to perform. Clasping at straws, a moment of inspiration or a product of fixation? The transcript of King George's famous war-time speech. I could sell it as some sort of 'meta' performance. It's famous for its stammering. I stammer. It was the only idea I had.

After my first performance they want it again. But this time Barry has an idea. Is he inspired by the recent showing of 'Educating Yorkshire' on Channel 4, or has he seen the innovative methods of King George's own therapist Lionel Logue? Or maybe Barry, like all aspiring musicians, just wants to lay down a sick beat. This time I'm to perform the piece listening to a rhythmic composition on Barry's headphones. Like magic, my speech becomes fluent, and I embellish this wondrous metamorphosis with musicality and melody. I knew what was going to happen, but the class didn't. They're stunned. Applause follows. Congratulations to me.

I came away from the class feeling lighter – and I couldn't pinpoint why. For the rest of the module I continued to stammer, but my experience of speaking was different. I had come into the module with a bone to pick with stammering. I had suffered at the hands of my stammer all year, struggling through practical exams that I felt ill equipped for. My stammer had been a burden, in my mind a key component of my inadequacies as a medical student.

In that class, I realized that what stammering *meant to me* had transformed. From being a heavy weight, to a musical device. From being something to be ashamed of and to hide, to something the group could focus on and analyze. It turned from something deeply personal, to something measurable and disposable. In this chapter of my life, my stammer had ceased to be the problem it once was. What my stammer meant to me, and others, had changed. And yet, besides the couple of minutes of speaking over a beat, my physical stammering had hardly changed at all. This really blew my mind.

I've had a few moments of clarity like this in my life, where it's felt like my experience of stammering would change forever and that would be it. Problem solved. Only, a few days later I would find myself back in the same old habits, having the same old feelings, struggling yet again with this stubborn stammering problem. Fortunately, I was about to stumble into an area of literature that would beautifully articulate the realization I had in that class. 'Narrative Therapy' ended up being the focus of my research project for the module and a key tool in my development as a person who stammers and as a doctor today.

So began my education into the social model of stammering. With it, a freedom to think creatively and positively about stammering. Using Narrative Therapy in a reflective journal led me to repeated journeying from thoughts in my head to ink on paper, and to a space for decision and action. A space to achieve clarity on the important things I wanted in my life and to discern how I spent my time. Crucially, it weaponized the social model of stammering to be brought into my everyday life, and located the power in me to bring about change. Over time, this approach has led to a life where I can better support myself, prioritize my needs, and make stammering a positive.

In this chapter, I want to introduce you to some of the brilliant ideas I found in Narrative Therapy. Using my own story, I want to bring these ideas to life. I'd like to challenge you, the reader, to think about stammering (and problems generally) in a new way – introducing an approach that has brought me enormous relief and energy. I believe that experiencing something for yourself is one of the most effective modes of learning, so throughout the chapter I have some exercises for you to think through. There are some technical terms in Narrative Therapy that can be challenging to understand. I've highlighted them in **bold** and given definitions in a glossary at the end of the chapter. If you are interested in Narrative Therapy, I've also added a reading list.

Narrative Therapy

Narrative Therapy helps people in an entirely novel way. It is built from social theory, so from the very philosophy it is based on, to the therapeutic practices it uses, Narrative Therapy is different from more behaviorally-oriented therapies. Narrative Therapy opens a door to see stammering from an alternative point of view, which for me offers the greatest opportunity for positive change.

I struggled for many years to understand myself as a 'stammerer'. As stammering began to swell up and overwhelm me as a teenager, my personhood and identity began to become obscured. I ceased to be a normal boy and began to be a stammerer. The tendency to label people with pathology is commonplace in the medical field. After all, if you have broken your leg or been bitten by a deadly snake, labelling things correctly is an essential ingredient to ensure swift diagnosis and prompt treatment. But under the label of 'a stammerer', or 'an anorexic', 'a refugee', 'a schizophrenic', where does the rest of your identity reside? Narrative Therapy calls the effects of this labelling a 'totalizing technique'; the process of internalizing events to be situated within a person, and thus restricting a person to a narrow and all-encompassing description of the self. It is from this place that a **problem-saturated narrative** is born – a story about yourself that revolves around a problem.

Narrative Therapy doesn't situate problems in people. Nor does it try to solve or cure a problem. Instead, it tries to improve our relationship with a problem. It considers how problems are produced in a social, cultural and political context. These problems are experienced principally in the form of stories. For Michael White and David Epston, the founders of Narrative Therapy, stories provide the framework on which we hang our everyday life. Stories help us make sense of the world – a thread linking events from an infinite amount of experiences into a meaningful sequence. We have numerous stories about ourselves and others – the story about ourselves at school, the story of us at work, the story of us as a performer or as a friend. The narratives we develop about ourselves come to define us and govern our lives in our thoughts, feelings, actions and imagination. The relationship between the narrative we develop and the life we lead can be thought of as a two-way affair. According to Jerome Bruner, just as Aristotle might say that art imitates life and Oscar Wilde might say that life imitates art, narrative imitates life and life imitates narrative. The stories of the past therefore bring meaning to the present and open the door to the stories of the future.

Exercise 1: Stammering as a problem

1. Consider what it would be like to stammer if everyone in the whole world stammered. What would everyday life look like? To what extent would stammering be a problem?

2. Stuttering is what you do trying not to stutter (Wendell Johnson). What do you think of this phrase? What are the conditions that make people not want to stammer?

Exercise 2: Problem-saturated narrative

1. How much do you think about stammering? (If you don't stammer, do you have a problem you think about a lot?)

2. Can you recount a story from your week where you have faced this problem? Write the story down or tell a friend/family member the story. What was the story like? How did you think, feel and behave in the story? What did others do?

3. If you can't think of a story now, keep an eye out for one in the next day or two, and pay close attention to what happens.

According to the Dulwich Centre, founded by Michael White, Narrative Therapy helps clients by enabling them to separate their lives and relationships from those stories they find impoverishing, assisting them to challenge the ways of life that they find subjugating, and encouraging persons to re-author their own lives according to alternative and preferred stories of identity. Stammering is different for everyone – everyone has different stories. At the beginning of the 'Arts in Healthcare' module, stammering featured heavily and negatively in my life's narrative. Narrative therapists would call this a '**problem-saturated**

narrative. Stammering was everywhere, never too far from my mind and a dominating character. Narrative Therapy gave me an opening to get away from such a problem-saturated narrative and find alternative and empowering stories.

The first step would be to start paying attention to my life's story - to figure out exactly what was going on to create such a 'problem-saturated narrative'. Next, I would need to '**deconstruct**' the stories I told, critiquing them by delving beneath the surface and developing a more useful and complex understanding. Then, looking forward, I could break from the problem-saturated narrative by finding rich and diverse moments for myself that I would record with depth and expression, to form paths to new empowering stories. To show you this process in action, I want to take you back to two seminars from my time as a student, where I was beginning to experiment with the narrative process.

Stammering is bad.
Stammering is ugly.
Stammering is failure.
Stammering is something to hide.
Stammering is something to be afraid of.
Stammering is not normal.

My story

Twice a week throughout my degree at university, we would have a seminar where we discussed a clinical case as a way to guide our learning. The final session of the week would be an opportunity to share our learning and discuss the critical points that were central to the case. Over the years, I began to resent this time of the week and would be filled with anxiety about sharing and reading.

One week was typical of the times before it, and with narrative in mind, I went into the seminar keen to observe what would unfold. I later reflected:

> "I began to explain to my peers the mechanism of how the cancers of the lung spread through the body. As I began to talk, and stammer through my explanation, I felt like I was losing my audience. People started to look down, stare into space, and when I finished, a resounding silence filled the room. The familiar feeling of failure swept over me. My stammer had yet again come in the way of success."

I decided to revisit this experience as part of my narrative approach. During the seminar I had observed my thoughts, feelings and behaviour around speaking and I had also monitored the sequence of events that had unfolded in the room. I challenged myself; what was it exactly that I failed at here? Ultimately this was a failure in communication, and I had come up with the familiar line – failure due to stammering.

As I started to **deconstruct** the story I had originally made, I began to uncover some significant holes. Had my stammer caused the failure in communication? On consideration, besides stammering I realized there were a lot of other factors that led me to communicate poorly in this instance. Had I found what I was saying particularly interesting? No. Was I particularly enthusiastic about the topic and willing to engage people? No. Was I even that knowledgeable about what I was saying? No. In fact, I realized that my preparations on the subject had been slim and I did not feel at all confident in the area I was talking about. I was struck by the realization that in the event of absolute fluency I would not have held the attention of the room either. In terms of narrative, I had re-authored my initial 'thin', one-dimensional and simple description of events into something much more complex and useful to me, a '**thick description**'.

As part of my reflection, I also questioned the intentions, beliefs and values that were leading me through the seminar. I had begun thinking in these terms following a brief experience in Cognitive Behavioural Therapy and reading about the Stammering Hexagon in John Harrison's *Redefining Stuttering*. I had never formulated these ideas into a reflection before. In these seminars, I observed that my main intention when speaking was to 'not stammer'. This intention filled my mind so much that it barely left any space to consider the substance of what I was talking about. Observing my thoughts and stories in other situations, I realized that my definition of success in a lot of speaking situations was based almost entirely around fluency. In each case, appraising the outcome as 'good' or 'bad' depended on whether I could get my words out fluently or not. Here a key belief of mine was brought to light – that fluency equalled success.

I turned my thoughts to the broader societal, cultural, ideological pressures that had formed my fluency-centric mind: the conditions that made stammering a problem in my life. I lived in a world that valued first impressions and superficial appearances. People's opinions of me were very important to me. This world valued achievement and success over much else. Success was linked to being confident, articulate and fluent. To be a good doctor you had to be fast, efficient, and silky smooth.

The following week I changed my plan for the seminar. I decided I would study hard and ensure I could come to class with an area in which I was passionate, informed, and well-rehearsed. I also decided that since it was a given I would stammer, rather than worry about it, I would place my entire focus and energy that morning in the science I was to discuss. I would depend on the speaking techniques developed at a London City Lit speech therapy course to get through my blocks and forget about stammering altogether. The results were striking. For the first week in years, I enjoyed myself in a seminar. I spoke, and stammered, with clarity and depth and expression. And people listened. People listened! I had found a **unique outcome** - evidence contrary to the problem saturated narrative. In this case, evidence that failure was due to stammering was inaccurate. This opened the door to a new narrative - stammering, with the right preparation, could lead to effective communication. I decided to record this story down and **thicken** the description as much as possible. So began the start of a New Approach, a story that I would take forward and begin to experiment with.

Exercise 3: Unique outcomes

Using the same problem you thought about in Exercises 1 and 2, do you have a moment recently that was different to the normal problem-saturated narrative? Record it in a story.

Try to capture the:

- Action: including describing the people, the place and the actions in the story. What happened, in what sequence, involving which characters?

- Consciousness: How did you/people feel, know and think? What were your intentions, desires, values and beliefs?

There were some key learning points I made at this initial stage of using Narrative Therapy. I realized that stammering and having a problem with stammering were not the same thing. Here I had two examples in the same situation that both involved stammering but had two completely different stories. The respective stark similarities and differences of the two stories highlighted how powerful I was in developing my own stories. The interpretative step had been made clear. I realized I had a choice in how I reacted to my stammer and I had a choice in how I approached all of the other factors that led to effective communication. I realized that the problem was not the problem. My problem was having a problem with the problem. I felt empowered by this realization. I had uncovered a power to develop my own stories. I think only people who stammer will appreciate how momentous this was! In those moments of stammering I feel utterly powerless, helpless, almost stuck in time. This sense of power and agency was a new feeling and a profound realization.

I also realized that at the heart of my problematic responses to my stammer was a fluency-centric mentality. In just one instance, where I had changed my intention from speaking fluently to speaking honestly, I was able to transform my experience of speaking.

By deconstructing my stories, I was able to develop an understanding of the beliefs, intentions and values that I held which supported unhelpful reactions to stammering. Further, I could develop an understanding of the social conditions from which these beliefs, intentions and values had formed. Social theorists believe that we live according to 'social norms', social rules that we inherit from our surroundings – institutions, family, the media, and culture. We subconsciously take on these rules and employ them without realizing – judging ourselves according to them constantly. Historically these rules might be 'thin girls are beautiful', 'black people don't have the capacity to vote', 'homosexuals are a lesser form of human', or 'stammering is unacceptable'.

Without insight into how we inherit these rules/norms, it's easy to believe these ideas to be truths of the world. But with a critical approach, it's possible to see these rules instead as artefacts from the societies we are born into. Narrative Therapy gave me a sounding board to realize the presence of these social norms and 'presumed truths' and to challenge them rather than internalize them. The continued insights I made had a hugely liberating effect on me – by realizing what these rules had been installed in me – as my beliefs, intentions and values, I could decide whether to follow them or challenge them. In unique outcomes I would look for exceptions to the norms. I was surprised at how often these came. I realized that a lot of the time others did not hold my beliefs. I also realized I had the capacity to think differently and develop my own set of rules that might break from 'social norms' but could still work for me.

All of a sudden, I had the potential to be a good doctor *with* a stammer. In choosing to forge my own path, and break from the status quo, my actions could have political weight. An action of non-avoidance or voluntary stammering was a positive stand against an ableist society that encourages conformity and marginalizes the 'sick' and 'weak'. To a social media generation that parades the glossy and pristine, my stammer could be a beautiful thorn. Depicting a stammer in these terms can bring fire to the belly and energy to the voice when motivation and self-belief have dwindled.

> "Modern psychology has a word that is probably used more than any other word in modern psychology. It is the word maladjusted. But I say to you, my friends. There are certain things in our nation and in the world which I am proud to be maladjusted. I never intend to become adjusted to segregation and discrimination. I never intend to become adjusted to religious bigotry. I never intend to adjust myself to economic conditions that will take necessities from the many to give luxuries to the few. I never intend to adjust myself to the madness of militarism, to self-defeating effects of physical violence... Through such maladjustment, I believe that we will be able to emerge from the bleak and desolate midnight of man's inhumanity to man into the bright and glittering daybreak of freedom and justice. My faith is that somehow this problem will be solved." Martin Luther King Jr., 1963 WMU speech.

The future

Stammering openly is Honesty
Stammering is Challenging, which can lead to Opportunity
Stammering is Authentic
Stammering can be Humbling
Stammering is Human

From this early experience I made a few intentional changes about the way I approached speaking situations. Since my problem with stammering had long been defined by avoidance, I decided to change what I valued in communication. Avoidance was supported by valuing fluency and I was keen to break with this habit, so rather than focus on fluency I switched my attention to communicating honestly and authentically. Every day I would look out for situations when I successfully did so, however small or benign the situation was, and I would pick these as unique outcomes. Examples: asking for a bus ticket without word substituting; introducing myself on the ward without using a filler word; holding eye contact with a person in a kiosk. I'd then thicken these stories up with detail. With every story, I grew further and further away from the problem-saturated narrative I had lived out just months before. Instead new paths were forming.

I soon discovered how a term like 'stammering aesthetic' could apply to me. I had heard the term at a BSA conference but failed to truly understand how it would take shape in my life. By using techniques, like voluntary stammering and self-advertising, with an open mind and a playful attitude, I found positive experiences of stammering were plentiful. By intentionally logging them down, I had a method of capturing it all, and as the pages and chapters unfurled, evidence grew to support this new method.

For me, Narrative Therapy offers a marriage of the medical and social approaches to stammering. The social approach is perhaps limited in that it can frame people as passive recipients of social structures and pressures, and risks pointing the finger at the world and willing it to change – an ideal approach but no short-term, pragmatic solution. The medical approach risks placing pathology in people and reinforcing negative stereotypes by normalizing medical societal standards. Might Narrative Therapy be a bridge between the two? Narrative Therapy has an individualized approach, facilitating individual change. However, there is a focus directed outwards at the social, empowering individuals to be liberated from dominant societal understandings, to select systems of knowledge that nourish and support rather than scourge and subordinate.

Narrative Therapy has been the recipient of reasonable criticism. Its post-structuralist, social constructionist roots are a radical departure from the therapies before it. Critiques of these philosophical standpoints apply both to Narrative Therapy's theory and practice. A subject still in its infancy, Narrative Therapy remains to be properly 'tried and tested' in speech therapy. Large clinical studies remain to be conducted providing evidence for its efficacy and long-term effectiveness. The nature of Narrative Therapy makes such studies difficult, though not impossible, to carry out.

In spite of these criticisms, my contention is that Narrative Therapy is vital for stammering. It offers a critical opportunity for the social model of stammering to be distilled, weaponized, and activated in individuals who might live out these ideas. In a field that has long been dominated by the medical model, Narrative Therapy can bring about much-needed change. Change that might precipitate in an individual's life, bringing congruence, authenticity and self-belief, but also in surrounding communities. My hope is that such an approach might galvanize people who stammer to step past simply advertisement, and stride into advocacy.

> "The radical, committed to human liberation, does not become the prisoner of a 'circle of certainty' within which reality is also imprisoned. On the contrary, the more radical the person is, the more fully he or she enters into reality so that, knowing it better, he or she can better transform it. This individual is not afraid to confront, to listen, to see the world unveiled. This person is not afraid to meet the people or to enter into dialogue with them. This person does not consider himself or herself the proprietor of history or of all people, or the liberator of the oppressed; but he or she does commit himself or herself, within history, to fight at their side." Paulo Freire, *Pedagogy of the Oppressed.*

Glossary

Problem-saturated narrative: A narrative that is reduced to a single theme. Instead of containing multiple and diverse voices and experiences, a problem-saturated story lacks complexity, forming into a singular narrative. Under a problem-saturated narrative, a person who stammers moves through life seeing a story filled with stammering. Whether it's asking for stamps at the post office, going on a date with a new partner or making an announcement at work, stammering is the key character. This recurring narrative constrains life and blinds the person to all events outside of this dominant singular narrative – they ignore, trivialize or don't notice the events outside of this understanding.

Thin description: A simple, one-dimensional account of events.

Deconstruction: The term originates from the work of philosopher Jacques Derrida, where it was used to explore of the 'slipperiness of meaning'. At the heart of Derrida's work is a critique of the relationship between text and meaning; that words only carry meaning when thought of in relation to other words. Meaning is therefore not essential, but dependent on context, history and climate. More simply, in Narrative Therapy deconstruction allows us to challenge the meaning making of our stories. Just as a fish is the last to discover water, deconstruction helps to expose the hidden assumptions or 'presumed truths' that lie within our stories, piercing our original 'thin' stories to find inconsistencies which prompt further questioning. By deconstructing stories we're able to appreciate how stories are constructed, or importantly simply realize that they are constructed in the first place. Under deconstruction a piece of narrative transforms from being an absolute depiction of your life, to just one of many other possible interpretations, one that is moulded and formed in an environment governed by geography, politics, culture and personnel (Freedman & Combs, 1996). With this understanding, a person who stammers is free to be curious and experiment with the way he/she comes to make meaning with the world.

Unique outcomes (innovative moments): Moments that fit outside of the problem saturated narrative. They encompass a wide range of experiences, from times where you've experienced a familiar situation without facing the problem, times when you approached the problem in a different way to moments when you understood the problem in a completely different way. The unique outcomes, or innovative moments form openings into new stories.

Thickening the plot: Creating rich, multilayered and varied stories. This provides an opportunity to give consideration to those memories or plots to which we want to ascribe particular meaning. When I came across a unique outcome in my day, I would later take time to remember the experience with as much detail, colour, and humour as possible and keep a record of it in my diary. Joining unique outcomes together over time thickens the plot further and begins a journey into a New Approach.

Reading list

Besley, T. (2009). Foucauldian influences in narrative therapy: An approach for schools. *The Journal of Educational Enquiry*, 2(2).

Bruner, J. (2004). Life as narrative. *Social Research: An International Quarterly*, 71(3), 691-710.

Carr, A. (1998). Michael White's narrative therapy. *Contemporary Family Therapy, 20*(4), 485–503.

Combs, G. & Freedman, J. (2012). Narrative, poststructuralism, and social justice. *The Counseling Psychologist, 40*(7), 1033–1060.

Freedman, J. & Combs, G. (1996). *Narrative Therapy: The Social Construction of Preferred Realities.* New York: WW Norton.

Morgan, A. (2000). *What is Narrative Therapy? An Easy-to-Read Introduction.* Adelaide: Dulwich Centre.

White, M. (1998). *Narrative Therapy.* Adelaide: Dulwich Centre.

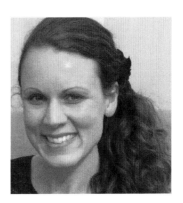

I chose this photo as I was out on a ship at sea and I'm generally pretty happy when I'm near the water.

Bella's secret

Sarah Michelle Wilkinson

Bella had a secret. A secret she wanted to hide, so it remained a secret forever.

Bella's secret wasn't so easy to keep. She didn't want to talk about it, but all the same she knew that people noticed it.

It wasn't that she really, really, hated it. It was just that sometimes she simply wanted to ignore it for a bit. Pretend that it wasn't there. Pretend she was just Bella, without the secret.

When Bella's parents took her to someone who said they could help her manage the secret better, Bella was quite frightened. She really did want the secret to be a bit more... in the *background*... But Bella didn't want someone asking lots of questions.

Bella was surprised, when her parents took her to the appointment, that it wasn't scary at all. The kind lady asked all about the secret, and Bella told her. When the lady told Bella that a lot of people have a secret just like hers, Bella was very happy.

The lady also told Bella how important it was to make her secret a bit less secret. Bella thought this sounded very good.

And so Bella started to let her secret become less secret.

Every day, the secret grew smaller, and Bella felt a little bit lighter...

And lighter...

Until Bella's secret was so much smaller and lighter that it wasn't a secret at all, any more. It was just a part of Bella.

Looking back, looking forward

Sam Simpson

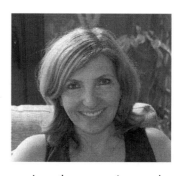

In my therapy room in my garden
– such a peaceful space for reflection.

"How do we recognise the shackles that tradition has
placed on us?
For if we can recognise them, we are able to break them."

Frank Boas

The social model of disability had largely passed stammering by until this decade. Despite this slow start, we are gaining ground and an international community of stammering activists has emerged: blogging, vlogging, producing works of art, networking, campaigning and creating new, empowering understandings of stammering. In this chapter, I want to look back and plot my experience of this progressive cultural movement. I will also look forward and consider the challenges and opportunities this radical development presents for the role and scope of future stammering research and therapy. Interwoven are my reflections, insights and ongoing learning from my engagement with the social model of disability.

I will start by looking back... to October 2016 and a blog post I wrote entitled 'Stammering activism and speech-language therapy: An inside view' for DidIStutter.org, reproduced here with their consent:

"Was I really dysfluent...?" the presenter whispered to her colleague as she sat back down in her seat. An innocent question on the face of it... a question, I found troubling, however, in the context in which I overheard it – the presenter was a (fluent) speech and language therapist returning from the podium having given a highly-polished presentation at an international stammering conference. The empathic part of me reached out to the fact that speech and language therapists are human and also fall prey to society's worship of 'fluency' and pervasive narratives around 'excellence'. However, the question also struck me as insidious. A speech and language therapist...?

At an international stammering conference...? Wasn't this of all places a forum where being dysfluent was totally OK...?

From a young age I've had a strong sense of social justice, and the principles of respect and value for each individual have been highly important to me. Feeling disrespected or seeing others be disrespectful has always made me angry. Fast-forward to my final year of postgraduate training to become a speech and language therapist here in the UK, when a tutor recommended a book that had just been published: 'Mustn't Grumble' - a controversial collection of short stories and poems reflecting the varied facets of disabled women's experience. How little did I know that it would challenge everything I was learning to the core.

Through this text, I uncovered a deep connection with the radical ideas underpinning the disabled people's movement. The clearly articulated and angry stories of oppression and exclusion taught me that, from a social model perspective, people aren't disabled because they have an impaired body, mind or means of communication, but because society places structural, environmental and attitudinal barriers in their way. Viewing disability as a civil rights and justice issue rather than a medical or therapeutic one resonated deeply – there was something refreshing, raw and alive about the social model and its open invitation to engage in a dialogue about difference that extended beyond the focus of loss and adjustment. However, it represented a direct challenge to the influential medical model, which has traditionally shaped the institutions within which speech and language therapists are trained and generally work in the UK and which perpetuates the historical focus on 'deficit' and the need for 'therapeutic intervention' by 'trained, expert practitioners'. As a therapist-in-training, it was unsettling to discover the extent to which the social model contested the fundamental principles upon which therapy is based. Furthermore, as much therapeutic practice has traditionally focused on 'normalisation' and the 'reduction or eradication of difference', the social model revealed an intrinsic paradox; that the narrow focus of restoration therapy can only serve to reinforce and reaffirm social norms and stigma rather than acting as a vehicle through which these prevailing norms can be challenged and renegotiated.

As a speech and language therapist I've worked in both the fields of stammering and brain injury. I believe my approach to therapy has benefited greatly from the cross-fertilisation of different ideas, theories and practices within these two fields. I was fortunate from early in my career to have ready access to forward-thinking aphasia therapists committed to engaging with the social model more actively. Through their pioneering work, many people with aphasia have been given a voice and role in defining the lived experience of aphasia and evaluating therapy services here in the UK. This has prompted a call for the focus of therapy to broaden and address the role that self-identity, society and social stigma play in making the processes of living with aphasia more challenging.

In contrast, I've been intrigued by how slowly the social model has been embraced within the stammering community. Indeed, the powerful influence of the medical model is still very apparent – as demonstrated by the growing interest in the neuroanatomical basis of stammering and fluency shaping approaches for young children that currently dominate conference programmes. However, in the spirit of client autonomy and choice, no matter how dominant, the medical model is only one lens through which stammering and stammering therapy can be viewed. The social model clearly illustrates how prevailing norms, language and stereotypes can go unchallenged, become internalised and, therefore, self-oppressive. This is of particular relevance to stammering and enables us to reconsider and re-define where the 'problem' of stammering is located.

I'm delighted to see a growing number of people who stammer engaging directly with the disability activist movement: The Did I Stutter? Project, members of the British Stammering Association (BSA) and the Employers Stammering Network (ESN) to name but a few. Also, that stammering therapists are starting to engage in these conversations too. Positioning the stammering therapy discourse within the broader disability discourse offers a means of revising and extending the boundaries of thinking about stammering and stammering therapy.

So, what might this mean for stammering therapists? Naturally, I can only speak from personal experience. The following is a reflection on how engagement with the social model has enriched and informed my philosophy of therapy and how I embody theory in practice.

The social model has encouraged me to embrace ideas that promote thinking against the grain. It's pushed me to critically examine my attitudes, beliefs and assumptions about otherness, difference and disability and how these have been shaped over time. This in turn has challenged me to actively reflect on and question my personal motives for the work that I do and to articulate my philosophy of therapy more clearly and transparently with clients. For me, stammering therapy is about reducing social- and self-oppression through the recognition, removal or negotiation of structural, physical and attitudinal barriers in order for people to live choice-fully and stammer openly, confidently and without shame.

To this end, the social model has taught me the importance of transforming social relationships and power dynamics, which involves being willing to get out of the therapy room and into the real-world context. I'm currently involved in co-developing and -facilitating a corporate training programme in conjunction with a business leader from the Employers Stammering Network (ESN) and therapists from City Lit. The ESN is an organised initiative, which together with the British Stammering Association (BSA), is working to change society's understanding of and attitudes towards stammering in the UK workplace. Following the success of a pilot project last year, we are now rolling out a more extensive programme of workshops for employees who stammer, managers and HR departments.

The social model has taught me the power of language and to be mindful of how I talk about and frame stammering. I consistently avoid using the binary oppositions 'bad-good' that place stammering on the negative pole and reinforce fluency as the gold standard in an ongoing commitment to not reinforce ableism. I also avoid framing stammering as 'a defect', 'impediment' or 'disorder' and openly question others' use of such language. In addition, the social model has taught me to respect personal language preferences in others (e.g. person-first or identity-first language, such as 'person who stammers' or 'stammerer'), the political stance that language of identity can represent and the perils of unquestioningly applying a broad linguistic standard, such as PWS.

Engaging clients in conversations about the contrasting ways difference is understood in society and the different ways stammering can therefore be defined is central to my approach to therapy. I frequently witness how liberating an understanding of the social model can be as it shifts the focus away from 'what is wrong with me' to critically examining 'what is wrong with the broader system in which I live'. Being explicit and transparent about my philosophy of therapy also enables clients to make more informed decisions about what they feel might be helpful at a particular point of time. There is no 'one size fits all' in stammering therapy, so offering a range of approaches and recognising that people's therapy preferences change over time affords greater client autonomy. I balance idealism with realism; whilst the growing number of radical stammering communities are re-visioning stammering and the future, it will inevitably take time for this important work to impact the day-to-day reality for everyone who stammers. Therapy, therefore, involves the delicate balancing act of offering access to these radical communities and their vision whilst also working from where people are at. That said, the social model has also taught me greater humility, an appreciation that many people live well with stammering outside of therapy and to therefore not view the need for therapy as automatic.

I have found that introducing people to research into stigma and self-stigma [see Michael Boyle's chapter] as well as the concept of internalised oppression offers a different way of bringing about changes in attitude. Additionally, introducing people to stammering activism and dysfluency pride offers people an opportunity to explore and discover new identities and communities. Social media is a powerful mechanism for bringing people together, so I try to stay current and signpost diverse resources and communities via Twitter and Facebook. Additionally, in keeping with the belief that the 'personal can become political' I regularly encourage people to blog, vlog, write articles, get involved in student and therapist training as well as co-presenting at conferences. A number of clients have since gone on to campaign more actively through organised public speaking events, the production of documentaries and the creation of peer groups and other political platforms for people to join together as a collective and challenge prevailing negative attitudes and misconceptions about stammering.

I'm so very grateful that a book recommendation opened my eyes to the social model and the disabled people's movement so early in my career. It has affirmed the importance of staying open to a plurality of ideas and theories as well as the value of exploring views that deviate from conventional thought and practice. While this has resulted in a career path that hasn't always been straightforward to navigate, it's undoubtedly shaped a path that has been more colourful, creative and enriching as a result.

Returning to the therapist I overheard at the international stammering conference... to me, what remains so deeply insidious in their query is what has not yet been questioned and what, therefore, remains out of awareness and unexamined. This strikes me as perilous not only for the individual therapist concerned, but, if representative of the majority, for stammering therapy and the stammering community at large.

What stands out to me as I re-read this blog post a number of years later is my anger and my passion. The poet David Whyte, in his book *Consolations: The Solace, Nourishment and Underlying Meaning of Everyday Words*, describes anger as the deepest form of compassion and the purest form of care illuminating what we wish to protect and are willing to hazard ourselves for. This speaks to the part of me that cares deeply about the way stammering is commonly understood and talked about, both in professional contexts and the public domain, as this has a powerful influence over the frames of reference adopted by people who stammer themselves.

In raising these concerns more publicly in recent years, I have thrown a number of sizeable pebbles into the water – from presenting with Katy Bailey and St John Harris at the Oxford Dysfluency Conference in 2014; co-organizing the Stammering Pride and Prejudice Conference at City Lit with Rachel Everard and Carolyn Cheasman in 2016; to ensuring stammering pride has a platform at recent BSA conferences together with Katy Bailey, Iain Wilkie, Rachel Everard and Patrick Campbell. As naturally follows with pebble throwing, these conversations have made variably-sized splashes in both professional arenas and within the stammering community itself. It has been interesting to observe the myriad different reactions to this ongoing attempt to open up a dialogue about the relevance of the social model for stammering and their ripple effect.

On reflection, I haven't always prepared myself for the strength of people's reactions, particularly from my peers – the confusion, the anger and the criticism, such as questioning my professionalism for publicly talking about the potential for stammering therapy to be experienced as abusive. Zahari's words on page 72 resonate: "resistance is risky; you gain no friends when you expose the dystopic elements of society". In truth, being willing to put my head above the parapet and question some of the fundamentals of stammering therapy has been emotionally draining and lonely at times.

With hindsight, omitting to put on sufficient self-protection is surprising as many of my peers' responses mirrored my own feelings of professional destabilization when I first encountered the social model in the 1990s. Indeed, their anger has enabled me to reconnect with my own continued anger at feeling misled during my training by the lack of transparency regarding the foundational principles of speech and language therapy and how ingrained the medical model is to its central premises. I also recognize that anger can be symptomatic of fear and uncertainty. Was I was perhaps naïve to presume therapists would find questioning the medical basis of our thinking about stammering and stammering therapy immediately engaging, especially given the very gradual uptake of social model principles within the field? Maybe my initial hopes of bringing the discipline in line with disability theory were not wholly realistic? Was the pace of change I had hoped for overly-ambitious? What I certainly wasn't prepared for was the professional silence and inertia; having hoped to open up dialogue, debate and radical change, this left me feeling uncertain, vulnerable and exposed. In response, I lay quiet for a number of months to take stock. My withdrawal was perhaps a missed opportunity to reach out and follow up on people's more immediate responses.

What I recall from this perceived period of professional stillness was how elated I felt to see the social model capture the interest of changemakers within the stammering community. I was delighted to be invited by Iain Wilkie and Norbert Lieckfeldt to get involved in the Employers Stammering Network and, together with colleagues at City Lit, design and co-facilitate the pioneering 'Redefining Stammering at Work' workshop series. This collaboration enabled us to take therapy and disability theory directly into the corporate world, where we were in a prime position to influence attitudes and employment practice in a way I could never dream to achieve by staying in the safety of my therapy room.

Patrick Campbell's BSA blog post, 'What if we fight for our right to stammer?', offered another beacon of light during that period of darkness. It was wonderful to see someone else take up the social model mantle, engage openly with its foundational principles and ask important and challenging questions of the stammering community here in the UK. This was a timely tonic and the connection countered my growing feelings of professional isolation. Our early conversations sowed the seed for this book and led to our collaboration with Chris, whose writing 'across the pond' chimed with us both; another questioning voice resonating on the same sound wave. I value community and connection, so finding like-minded people, equally committed to challenging the assumed norms and narratives around stammering and therapy, felt liberating. Indeed, this collaboration has created a lively forum to engage with alternative models and critique the limitations of the social model which has been refreshing and stimulating; as well as an important personal reminder to stay open to other narratives and not become blinkered and narrow in my own view.

Despite my initial uncertainty and pessimism about interest in the social model, I am increasingly optimistic. Seeds need time to germinate, after all. In retrospect, I was primarily looking for change within the professional community. I wanted to hold stammering therapists to account for their slow engagement with the social model as compared to their peers working in the fields of aphasia, learning disability and autism. I was also keen to encourage deeper critical reflection on their potential contribution to the perpetuation of social norms and stigmatizing views on stammering. However, to my surprise, my early allies came from outside the profession. The new shoots and first signs of growth came from within the stammering community itself. A plethora of people here in the UK have begun to develop new and empowering meanings around stammering through art, photography, poetry, comic strips, literature, Ted-talks, public speaking competitions, and raps. The dynamic energy and tone of the 2016 BSA conference in Manchester, for example, was radically different – an open, unapologetic celebration of stammering through music, poetry, and improvisation to name but a few. The 'for one-night-only' Stammerband, composed entirely of people who stammer, played out an electric mix of songs related to stammering. The night featured rock anthems, such as 'My Generation' by The Who and 'You Ain't Seen Nothing Yet' by Bachman-Turner Overdrive. Powerful voices coming together in unison, demonstrating how stammering can be harnessed to enhance a message and break away from socially-conceived norms.

As stammering is being reclaimed as a different and valuable means of communication, a radical conversation around stammering gain is emerging (see Chris Constantino's chapter). This is revealing how the experience of stammering can shape and positively influence character traits, skill development and the quality of interpersonal relationships. Personal accounts have highlighted how stammering can foster personal courage, resilience, and resourcefulness. Moreover, stammering can offer a unique insight into the power of words, the subtlety of language, the importance of listening, the delicate shifts in nonverbal communication, and the different qualities of silence. It can also reveal the compelling power and intimacy of vulnerability and authenticity.

I am encouraged by observable changes in the language around stammering. Terms central to the social model, such as 'barriers', 'stigma' and 'discrimination' are now much more commonplace. Here in the UK, there are new policies around language and representation of stammering, spearheaded by Patrick Campbell during his time as a BSA trustee. Twitter is alive with people calling out public discrimination in the newspapers and on billboards, challenging mainstream ways of conceptualizing stammering to positive effect, as in the more recent campaign that led HSBC UK banking to change an advert that portrayed stammering in a negative way. A wonderful example of the potential, potency and collective force of *power with*.

Similarly, engagement in the development of public policy is now evident. Walter Scott is championing the discussion around oracy skills in education for young people who stammer. Claire Norman is leading the Stammerers Through University Consultancy (STUC) to develop awareness and support structures for university students and staff who stammer. The tireless work of the ESN is shaping UK employment attitudes and practice. Furthermore, Iain Wilkie's keynote presentation at the 2018 Joint World Congress in Japan has enabled links with international communities interested in extending the reach of this work. Thus, changes in the narrative around stammering are gradually being formalized and stitched more permanently into the fabric of our society.

Changes are also starting to take root professionally. Disappointingly, all the abstracts I submitted for the same stammering conference that inspired the 'Did I Stutter?' blog post three years later were declined; an indication that ongoing dialogue about the social model is not encouraged in some academic circles where scientific debate, neuroimaging, and impairment-based approaches continue to dominate. However, invitations to talk at Clinical Excellence Networks have gradually come in and further training courses via City Lit have made ongoing dialogue and debate possible. In keeping with the principles of the social model, these talks have embraced a collaborative approach. Presenting alongside Katy Bailey and Patrick Campbell has enabled the boundaries between therapist and people who stammer as holders of therapy knowledge to be extended and the dialogue enriched. Numbers to such events tend to be small and I am aware that we are often talking to the already converted; however, it is heartening to see that the community of stammering therapists embracing the social model is growing here in the UK.

Importantly, such forums have offered stammering therapists a cathartic platform to share the personal challenges of their work. Therapists have spoken openly of feelings of uncertainty and guilt about the mixed messages they may be perpetuating in therapy, especially when children and young people are transitioning to a more established stammering pattern; further heightened by feelings of responsibility under the weight of professional and parental expectations coloured by the dominant restorative narrative. The complexity and delicacy of conversations about hopes, expectations and therapy options are clear. These conversations take time and benefit from a more established therapeutic relationship that can be difficult to foster in the current climate of limited resources and pressure for throughput to meet exacting organizational targets.

In contrast, therapists have expressed excitement and liberation at being given the opportunity momentarily to put down established practices and expectations of stammering therapy services in order to creatively debate and share ideas on how these services could be reconfigured through a social model lens. The ripple effect of these conversations is gaining ground as therapists have trialled taking their innovative ideas out into their places of work. I have been approached for teaching materials to include in parent workshops to open up conversations about the way society understands difference and the influence this can have on how stammering is talked about at home. Therapists have experimented with shifts in practice, such as meeting with parents and discussing the pros and cons of working directly with the child ahead of meeting the child. Some therapists are working towards obtaining informed consent more transparently by sharing the full spectrum of viewpoints on therapy, so that parents can be more actively involved in deciding what therapy and when for their child. Other paediatric therapists are looking to collaborate with adult services so that more parents can meet adults who stammer in order to debunk myths and potentially stigmatizing views and gain a more informed understanding of the challenges and opportunities that stammering can bring. Increasingly, therapists are integrating the use of creative media (art, poetry, music, public speaking) to enable children, young people and adults to explore stammering pride and prejudice more directly – powerful examples of which have been shared informally over social media, or more formally through events such as the pioneering Hear in Hull 2017 City of Culture programme and the ISAD 2018 'My stammer' art exhibition.

As I survey the current landscape, it is remarkable to consider just how much momentum has been gained in recent years. Josh St Pierre has always argued that the real change needs to come from within the stammering community itself and it is evident that this movement is happening on an international scale. We have radical communities in the USA, such as the Did I Stutter? project that positively affirms dysfluent speech, as well as others, such as NYC Stutters who organize conferences exclusively for people who stammer to explore what can be learned from the disability rights movement about living in a fluent world. The 2018 Joint World Congress 'One World Many Voices: Science and Community' is representative of a move towards greater collaboration and integration between professionals and people who stammer. Similarly, the innovative 2018 conference 'Metaphoric Stammers and Embodied Speakers: Expanding the Borders of Dysfluency Studies' ambitiously set out to explore the experience and construction of stammering from the perspectives of literary/cultural analysis as well as stammering therapy and neurological research. This collaboration created a refreshing dialogue and exchange across these fields. It was liberating to move beyond conceptualizing dysfluency as a disorder to be treated, to exploring it as a unique form of communication that highlights the intricate relationship between speaking and being heard, vocal agency and cultural reception.

The world is now populated with many more radical voices redefining the narrative around stammering in an increasing number of different sectors. Contextually, these are riding on the wave of more widespread, fundamental social change. Of particular relevance is the cultural movement towards conceptualizing the world population as neurodiverse and consequently exhibiting a range of styles of social interaction. The Diversity and Inclusion discourse is gaining momentum and calling for the renegotiation of the narrative of disorder and a narrowly-defined norm. Similarly, Positive Psychology and the strengths movement are cultivating foreign consciousness, openness to difference, and the celebration of otherness and unique experience. These trends all seem to be converging to create the global environmental conditions for change towards greater authenticity, pride and respect.

So, looking forward... against this backdrop of profound social change, it is arguably time for speech and language therapy as a profession, and stammering researchers and therapists in particular, to reconsider their position and role. Central to this is the acknowledgement that, to date, the evolution of stammering therapy has been dominated by the medical model. Having shone our torch narrowly on one paradigm to define our terms of reference and scope of practice, the momentum for cultural change prescribes a professional and ethical imperative to extend the reach and consider different paradigms and their implications for the future of stammering therapy. This conversation is beginning. Chris and a small group of therapists who stammer took part in a pioneering panel discussion about current controversies in stammering therapy, including the social model, at the 2018 American Speech-Language-Hearing Association (ASHA) Convention. I hope this will lead to a greater recognition for the need to continue this dialogue at international stammering conferences. Such debates will naturally take us into new and unfamiliar territory; however, we risk becoming outdated if we do not consider the broader agenda for social change and what this means to the fundamentals of stammering therapy going forward.

Such a voyage calls for action at many levels. It calls for all educators to integrate the diversity agenda into the speech and language therapy curriculum in order for future stammering therapists to explore the philosophical underpinnings of their role and approach. Similarly, current therapists need open forums to re-examine their underlying values, role and scope of practice. We need more researchers willing to consider alternative conceptual frameworks to the medical model for future stammering research. For example, the social model of disability points to more widespread research into public awareness campaigns tackling stigma and stereotyping in addition to the development and coordination of robust information, education, and support programmes in schools, universities, and places of work as well as public services. This requires a balanced investment of resources focusing on tackling the day-to-day barriers experienced by young people and adults who stammer as well as neuroscientific developments and therapies for children. The social model also supports more meaningful collaboration with people who stammer to rethink the scope, focus, and role of future stammering therapy for children, young people and adults. This involves people who stammer becoming partners in research rather than onlookers being paid lip-service. We have seen tremendous advances in the fields of neuroscience and genetics in recent years, but I am not aware of any open, public debate about the broader social and ethical implications of this research. This dialogue seems critical if we want to avoid replicating the situation in Iceland where Down's Syndrome is rapidly disappearing following a 100% uptake of termination following developments in prenatal screening. What kind of society do we ultimately want to live in?

A world without stammering or a world that understands and gains from the experience of stammering?

A world that understands and gains from stammering is a world in which stammering is visible and upheld as a legitimate and valuable means of communication in its own right. Fundamental to this is representation. We need more healthcare practitioners and educators who stammer, more newsreaders and presenters, actors, artists, business leaders, politicians and international spokespeople. I can see a transitional role for speech and language therapists in terms of challenging social- and self-stigma to support people who stammer to fulfil their educational, professional, and personal dreams and potential. However, in the way that people with dialectal speech differences are no longer considered to have disordered speech and therefore in need of restorative speech and language therapy, I also hope for a future where stammering therapy will no longer be needed. Just as many charities now aim for 'extinction', effectively reaching a point where they are no longer needed, perhaps stammering therapists also need to aim for extinction? Maybe going forward our polestar is what needs to change in order for our services to become redundant? Whilst such a world is a long road ahead of us, it is nevertheless pleasing to see that we are now definitely on the path:

> "Pathmaker, your footsteps
> Are the path and nothing more;
> Pathmaker, there is no path,
> You make the path by walking."

> Antonio Machado

Further reading

Campbell, P. (2015, February 9). What if we fight for our right to stammer. Retrieved February 12th, 2019, from https://www.stammering.org/what-we-do/blog/what-if-we-fight-our-right-stammer

Constantino, C. (2016, October 1). Stuttering Gain. International Stuttering Awareness Day Online Conference. Retrieved February 12th, 2019, from http://isad.isastutter.org/isad-2016/papers-presented-by-2016/stories-and-experiences-with-stuttering-by-pws/stuttering-gain-christopher-constantino/

Finkelstein, V. (1993). Disability: A social challenge or an administrative responsibility? In J. Swain, V. Finkelstein, S. French, & M. Oliver (Eds), *Disabling Barriers – Enabling Environments*. London: Sage.

Keith, L. (1994). *Mustn't Grumble: Writing by Disabled Women*. London: The Women's Press.

Oliver, M. (1993). Disability and dependency: A creation of industrial societies? In J. Swain, V. Finkelstein, S. French, & M. Oliver (Eds), *Disabling Barriers – Enabling Environments*. London: Sage.

Oliver, M. (1996). A sociology of disability or a disablist sociology? In L. Barton (Ed.) *Disability and Society: Emerging Issues and Insights*. London: Longman.

Whyte, D. (2015). *Consolations: The Solace, Nourishment and Underlying Meaning of Everyday Words*. Langley: Many Rivers Press.

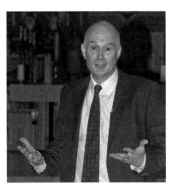

Taken at my EY leaving dinner at Southwark Cathedral, this photo reminds me how my relationship with public speaking has transformed over the years.

Finding our voices at work

Iain Wilkie

"Oh people look around you
The signs are everywhere
You've left it for somebody other than you
To be the one to care."

Jackson Browne

The boy stands at the lectern reading the morning's Old Testament lesson to the packed school assembly. He's a prefect, so he has to endure this agony every month.

He's frightened. He's frightened that he'll look stupid if he stammers in front of the whole school and of the teasing that will surely follow. So he swaps words that he can't say for others that he can. He leaves out the more difficult biblical names and replaces them with words like 'prophet' and 'elder'. Anything that looks like a potential stammering trap is neatly avoided.

From the outside, he sounds totally fluent. On the inside, he is a mess. Yet, no one else has the words in front of them and he gets away with it. He's done it before and he'll do it countless times again over the next 35 years. It's been another masterclass in stammering avoidance.

The man stands at the lectern reading the Old Testament lesson to the packed congregation at the memorial service in Southwark Cathedral for one of the firm's most esteemed partners.

This time he can't swap words because everyone else has them printed on the order of service. He'd worried beforehand that this might be the case. Nonetheless, his reading has started well. Then, all of a sudden, as if his head is an electric storm, his stammer shoots out across the congregation.

It's a very long block. Inside him it's mayhem. His stammering voice is bouncing back at him off the far wall of the cathedral. He needs three long breaths to get the word out. Eventually, the storm breaks and the word comes. He reads on and then returns in cathedral silence to his seat. He feels humiliated. He hasn't felt so lonely since his mother died when he was a boy.

The man sits quietly in his firm's leadership team meeting in the bright boardroom overlooking the Thames. He listens to a talk about becoming leaders in diversity and inclusion (D&I). He hears about gender, race, ethnicity, sexuality and much more. It is the right thing to do and he supports it all.

Yet in a business culture which prizes eloquent and efficient speech, he hasn't heard anything about language and speech differences, certainly not stammering – the demon which has held him down most in his career. He understands why. No one ever talks about stammering, especially him.

People who stammer want to hide it, not talk about it, while everyone else finds stammering awkward. There is a conspiracy of silence around stammering. He feels angry about it, even though he knows he's more to blame than most. After all, he knows about stammering; its embarrassment, its shame and how, even now as a senior partner, it sometimes still controls him.

From a bland study booth, the man calls the D&I manager. She listens with curiosity and then interest. They've not thought about stammering before, but if he'll commit to create a network they'll find some budget from somewhere to support it.

His pain stretches back 40 years.

Of course, he'll create a network. He'll lead it too.

The Ernst & Young Stammering Network is born.

One voice

> "If all this helps just one person to find their voice at
> work, it'll be worth it."
>
> The voice in my head.

It was now several months after I had launched the Ernst & Young (EY) Stammering Network. It was the only work-focused stammering network in the world and getting it going was proving much tougher than I had thought. There was no role model to follow. In the words of the Spanish poet Antonio Machado, I had to make the path forward myself:

> "Path maker, there is no path,
> You make the path by walking.
> By walking
> You make the path."

I put an announcement in the firm's 'Daily News'. It went to over 8000 people. With 1% of adults having a stammer, I reckoned there were around 80 people at EY in the UK in a similar boat as me. I was hopeful of at least 40 members within a year. However, the reality was that more than four months after launching, I was still my own little network of one. Yet, I was to discover later that the seeds of change had already germinated within some colleagues and that they would get in touch when the time was right for them. I just needed to keep showing that, when that time came, the network would extend a warm and secure welcome.

A few months later, Abid, a senior audit manager, contacted me asking if we would pay for him to attend an external stammering programme. Of course, I agreed. Then a couple of months later, Ricky, an undergraduate summer intern who stammered, joined me for a coffee. The following month, the three of us had a phone call together and Ricky said: "Hey guys, we've got ourselves a network!" It was music to my ears.

When Abid moved on from EY a couple of years later, we knew we would miss him, but also that our network group would survive. Gradually, one by one, our fragile group became stronger, growing in numbers, confidence, and impact. But why had it been so hard to get it started?

Workplace culture and stammering

> "No one dared
> Disturb the sounds of silence."
>
> Paul Simon

There are nearly 400,000 people of working age in the UK who stammer, yet it is a condition which remains largely hidden in the workplace. Employers are busy people and disability is surprisingly well down the list of diversity & inclusion (D&I) priorities. Consequently, in most working environments, no one speaks up for stammering.

Why is it difficult to be a person who stammers in the workplace?

There are uncomfortable challenges for employers when it comes to integrating stammering into the workplace. In particular, the irregular and unpredictable speech patterns of stammering challenge one of the prized beliefs about 'good communication'; namely that speech which is predictable and steady is desirable because it conveys competence and confidence, whereas speech with hesitations or repetitions suggests a lack of ability and nervousness. Of course, if we stopped and thought about it, we would agree that it is more valuable to listen to a speaker who stammers with great content than to a fluent presenter with weak content. Even the prophet Moses who described himself as "not eloquent" and "slow of speech and of a slow tongue" would have struggled to be heard in our 21st-century workplace where how we sound and speak invariably matters more than the substance of what we have to say.

Even now, it is common to mock stammering. One memorable moment for me was at a business social event recently when a former boss greeted me with "Hello, Iain WWWWWilkie", thinking everyone else would laugh. Instead, they looked to the floor in embarrassment as I explained to him that the world is moving on and so should he.

Stammering is often invisible to employers. Indeed, as people who stammer, we have been doing our best to keep it that way. This is due to the embarrassment, shame, and stigma associated with our 'imperfect' speech. After all, in working cultures where perfection is the expectation, why would we choose to advertise our imperfection?

As stammering only affects 1% of adults, for employers the economic case for action appears weak. Of course, with an almost endless list of differences, the answer ultimately lies in investing in an acceleration of the overall cultural transformation to acceptance and respect for all difference.

What does the research tell us?

Research indicates that people who stammer face prejudice and discrimination in the workplace. In 2014, when Dr Clare Butler interviewed people in the UK who stammer about their career experiences, she found that all of them believed that their stammer had negatively affected their career. Her work highlights how both employers and people who stammer allow speech to influence the jobs that they apply for and the chances of getting them. She showed how stammering can adversely impact career prospects and negatively affect the type of opportunities which are open to people who stammer. Butler identified systemic discrimination against stammering in the workplace and concluded that, "...the drive for sounding right... is exacerbating inequality, discrimination and social exclusion".

Furthermore, a paper by Hope Gerlach, Evan Totty and colleagues in 2018 found that both men and women who stutter earn approximately $7000 less than people of equivalent background, race and age in the United States for doing exactly the same job. This stammering pay gap is one that does not get reported in the media, but it is every bit as unacceptable as the gender, race and other pay gaps that do.

Cultural and physical barriers at work

Society's cultural barriers against people who stammer are prevalent in the workplace. A childhood of adverse reactions to our dysfluent speech inevitably leads to the withdrawal from many talking, reading, and social situations from an early age. This does not change when we enter the competitive world of work. In fact, it often increases due to the hierarchical structures and established communication protocols which reinforce fluency as an important attribute. Worse than that, dysfluency is regarded as a negative quality. These cultural barriers increase the pressure not to stammer, whether that is in low-profile conversations with our colleagues, high-profile sales presentations, or career-defining assessment centres.

Physical barriers are also prevalent. Examples include the requirement to communicate by telephone rather than in writing, the unforgiving exposure of the open-plan environment, or the increasing use of voice recognition technology by, for example, the banks.

Cultural and physical barriers often intertwine, particularly in early stage recruitment and promotion processes that are centred around efficiency: for example, telephone interviews where the only means of building a relationship between the candidate and the interviewer is through speaking and listening.

This is particularly tough for many candidates who stammer. It can also be hard on the interviewer because of the stress reaction a listener experiences when hearing stammered speech, especially if they have had no prior exposure.

Avoiding barriers by building barriers

"It ain't such a long drop, don't stammer don't stutter
From the diamonds in the sidewalk to the dirt in the gutter
And you carry those bruises to remind you wherever you go."

John Prine

For over 25 years, my response to these cultural and physical barriers was to develop my own ways of avoiding the painful consequences of crashing into them. Like most people who stammer, I built my own set of barriers especially for high-pressure situations where my stammer was more prevalent.

Avoidance techniques can be common for people who stammer at work, such as arriving late, missing meetings, avoiding giving presentations, not engaging in discussions, and perhaps even avoiding talking altogether. I often didn't speak up and withheld ideas for worry of being considered 'stupid' because I could 'not speak properly'. These self-imposed barriers seemed to work at the time, but every time I used them I was subtly and powerfully reinforcing my self-stigma of speaking with a stammer.

We have a working culture where employers' attitudes are consciously and unconsciously biased against stammering. People who stammer do not want to talk about it either. As Norbert Lieckfeldt, the talented former Chief Executive of the British Stammering Association, says, "There is a 'conspiracy of silence' around stammering at work". The net result is that people who stammer often do not fulfil our potential and employers and customers do not benefit from our full talents.

Positive developments: Diversity & Inclusion (D&I)

In spite of these troubling factors, we are lucky to live in an era where workplace assumptions and prejudices are being increasingly challenged. The inclusion and embracing of a greater diversity of people in the workforce is at the forefront of this movement. This is especially valuable in the UK, where 80% of the economy is service-oriented and based around people skills including our ability to communicate well with each other. For progressive employers, D&I also includes disability and health and, for an increasing number within that, stammering and speech.

Getting D&I right is much harder than it sounds, but for those organizations who achieve it the ethical and financial benefits can be huge. It can enable employers to recruit from wider talent pools, give a greater sense of engagement to people from minority groups and bring benefits from a variety of thinking and behavioural styles.

Taking chances

> "Sometimes you'll never be ready
> and you just have to go for it."
>
> Ed Balls

First chance: Going for it

The man is tired and happy. He'd got up early to be interviewed on the BBC's Radio 5 Live Breakfast show. It had gone well.

It's now early evening and he's in Westminster Hall in the Houses of Parliament where, over the centuries, many of our society's political and social changes have been born.

The man is nervous and excited. He's got a speech to give and he's taking a chance by publicly launching something new and untested. Yet his heart tells him these are risks worth taking. It's been over 40 years now. He hears his name announced and his heart is booming. His voice fills the void of expectant silence created by the one hundred guests. He attempts a little joke. They laugh. It's going to be OK.

He's launching the first national network in the world for employers who recognize stammering as a workplace issue. The evening is both hectic and serene. The Employers Stammering Network is born.

Early days for the Employers Stammering Network (ESN)

Created as part of the British Stammering Association (BSA), the ESN's vision is "to create a culture where people who stammer can achieve our full career potential". Alongside my knowledgeable ESN Co-Chair, Norbert Lieckfeldt, and myself were a dedicated and diverse group. Within a year of launching, and helped by a superb effort from Leys Geddes (former BSA Chair) and with terrific support from Ed Balls (former Government minister), the ESN had attracted several large employers to join us as members. Global giants such as Accenture, Citi, DHL, EY, HSBC, KPMG, Lloyds Bank, M&G, RBS and Shell were amongst them. The ESN planned to support the member organizations by sharing best practice; for example, encouraging stammering awareness activities, advising human resources and recruitment teams, and briefing line managers.

We quickly succeeded in raising the profile of stammering at work and were even recognized with a number of awards. Not everything went to plan, though. Over time, we became increasingly concerned that, in spite of strong employer membership growth, very few people who stammer were actually coming forward in the member organizations. Consequently not enough people were benefitting I knew from my EY experience that it would be slow, but had not anticipated that it would be this slow.

Then we got a lucky break.

Second chance: The social model

In July 2014, Norbert invited me to join him for a day at the Oxford Dysfluency Conference and, after listening to interesting sessions on brain structure and therapy techniques, we chose a new subject for the next session. Led by Katy Bailey, St John Harris and Sam Simpson, the title was curious: 'Stammering and the Social Model of Disability: Challenge and Opportunity' and, as it turned out, so was the substance.

It was radical stuff. The courageous presentation challenged the underlying principle of the conference that dysfluency needs to be better understood so that everyone can talk more fluently – or, in other words, that stammering is a problem that needs to be fixed. In contrast to this time-honoured belief and in front of a packed room, they were suggesting that dysfluency and stammering are not the problem at all. On the contrary, the problem lies in society's deeply-held belief that fluency is right and stammering is wrong. They argued that stammering is perfectly acceptable; indeed, it can even be seen as a desirable way of speaking. I had never heard anything like it! I lived and worked in a world which always assumed that stammering was a weakness. The question-and-answer session afterwards was lively as the new ideas were constructively challenged and old assumptions were stoically defended.

I was excited by the potential link to the workplace. The social model, with its acceptance of impairments and recognition of the importance of barriers, aligned tightly with the D&I model. Now we had something tangible that we could take to employers that could help change their attitudes towards stammering. The big question was how?

The personal therapist and the corporate accountant: An unlikely collaboration

Having approached Sam at the Oxford Dysfluency Conference, we started discussions about teaming up to bring the social model into the workplace for people who stammer. Initially, this took the form of a series of workshops.

The reality of bringing our two professions together to translate the theoretical social model into practical and sustained change for people who stammer at work was exciting. It was also more complex than I had anticipated. Our goals were perfectly aligned, but there was a big gap between how our worlds of personal therapy and large firms operate. It was the difference between personal and organizational perspectives, long- and short-term horizons and different success criteria. Nonetheless, our commitment to our overarching purpose meant that we got there.

The design model for the 'Redefining Stammering at Work' workshop programme was a series of three workshops piloted by the EY Stammering Network over a 5-month period in 2015. I attended as a participant. I learned how my relationship with my stammer was still being influenced by the culture at work, how it affected my stammering behaviour, the choices I made about being covert or overt about my stammer and the actions I could take going forward to achieve sustained change. Fellow stammering colleagues achieved similar benefits. The numbers attending grew during the course of the programme as its reputation spread. As the programme sponsor, I was thrilled with the outcomes and the financial pay-back for EY was amazing.

The extensive thinking invested in developing the workshops acted as the foundation for much of ESN's development activity over the next few years. In particular, the combination of the therapy and accountancy professional standards set the tone of a high-quality ESN experience with the intent to help deep change for individuals and sustained cultural change for employers.

Establishing the consistent quality benchmark was also important because ESN was diversifying in its activities and the range of people getting involved. Subsequent activities have included an ambitious pilot mentoring programme, workshops for employers, themed events and much more. The people involved now come from a wide range of employers, including small business owners and the self-employed.

Many voices

> "Never doubt that a small group of thoughtful committed citizens can change the world; indeed it's the only thing that ever has."
>
> Margaret Mead

Successful delivery of the workshop programme in 2015 and subsequent years played a key role in building a community of change-makers for stammering at work. Attendees would return to their employers feeling inspired to lead change and carrying the message 'It's OK to Stammer at Work'. This tag-line is for everyone: establishing acceptance by the 1% of us who stammer, and gaining acceptance by the 99% of colleagues who don't.

These change-makers, or Champions as we call them, work with their employers' culture, aligning their stammering activities to support the D&I goals of their own organization. Champions may form their own in-house networks, speak up publicly and become visible role models. Equally, they can be quiet leaders creating sustained change in the ways that they know can succeed within their own working culture. By mid-2018 ESN had over 40 Champions in its network.

This leadership-centred strategy has been more effective than our initial focus on attracting large organizations. Its ripple effect has also enabled many more people to benefit from ESN's activities. We now hold back from attracting more employers to join until they are ready.

Developing confidence

It can be lonely if you are the only person who stammers where you work, and from the beginning we built an informal ESN support network. This core network provides a welcoming and supportive environment for anyone interested in meeting others navigating stammering at work. Our first meeting attracted four people. Having grown one person at a time as its reputation spread, this community now numbers hundreds. It brings multiple benefits: allowing stories and successes to be shared, new friendships made and budding Champions to develop. Its diversity and inclusiveness are core to its effectiveness for individuals and employers.

At the core of the ESN's growth has been an openness to engage in courageous conversations with all people who stammer. Whether someone is a general in the army or a recent school leaver, one of our values is that it is the quality of how we connect personally with each other that determines the changes that we can achieve. When someone finds the courage to come forward to talk about their stammer, sometimes for the first time in their lives, they need to be met with empathy and a listening ear. Helen Carpenter, ESN's highly impactful manager from 2015, is particularly skilled in this area. Many people who stammer have benefited from Helen's welcoming conversations and some have subsequently become Champions themselves.

Employer networks

Reflecting its diverse personalities, the EY Stammering Network (EYSN) has become a creative hub of ideas and activity. With May Breisacher to the fore, recent publicity campaigns and working themes have focused on Strengths, the Stammering Iceberg, and being Unique – 'One in a Hundred'. Indeed, working with Engaging Minds, both EYSN and the ESN, have explored the work-related strengths that people who stammer typically develop as a consequence of a life journey with a stammer. Strengths which were common amongst a majority of the participants were high levels of empathy, listening, creativity and resilience. Such attributes are often valuable to employers. They can also enable people who stammer to be highly effective communicators.

A recent idea has been the 'Stammering Challenge', where colleagues who do not stammer are invited to voluntarily stammer during their working day. These ideas have helped to attract new members and allies as well as to raise awareness. They are also freely shared with other organizations through the ESN, including with non-ESN members.

The ESN acts as the umbrella and connector for several in-house employer stammering networks which it has helped to develop. These include the Defence Stammering Network (DSN) for both military and civilian personnel and the UK Civil Service Stammering Network, launched nationwide and across numerous departments. A new and exciting development in 2017 was the launch of the ESN's first regional network in Bristol showing the adaptability of the ESN's core employer network model

Working with the 99%

Our early recognition of the leading role played by employers in changing workplace culture was the reason we called ourselves the 'Employers' Stammering Network'. It overtly recognizes that the 99% of adults who are fluent hold the key to cultural change towards stammering at work.

The ESN's role includes helping educate allies within the 99% to understand stammering, and to help them attract, develop and retain stammering talent. Several ESN services have been developed specifically for employers. These include workshops for managers of people who stammer developed by Norbert and Rachel Everard of City Lit and the ESN's highly popular 'Understanding Stammering – A Guide for Employers'. This was written by Leys Geddes and subsequently expanded by Helen Carpenter with the support of the Employers Network for Equality & Inclusion (ENEI).

50 million voices

> "For the rest of the time that you're given,
> Why walk when you can fly?
> High"

> Mary Chapin Carpenter

Eight years have now passed since founding the EY Stammering Network and six years since launching the ESN. It feels timely to reflect on how far the cause of stammering at work has progressed, and where we may be headed next. I am absolutely thrilled that many hundreds of people who stammer have already benefited from our work, in addition to their families and employers.

Underpinning this have been the inclusive principles of the social model and their practical application aligning tightly with the values of D&I in the workplace. For over 150 employers this has resulted in greater awareness and support for stammering. Several employers now have their own stammering networks.

Looking forward

Although it will be a bumpy ride, the world's economy and its talent pool are likely to globalize further – and consequently D&I will become an even more important factor as organizations strive for success. Our opportunity is to work with these changes to help many more employers understand the benefits of supporting stammering at work. Can we take it?

In July 2018, I presented to the World Stuttering and Cluttering Congress in Hiroshima, Japan, on 'Redefining Stammering at Work'. The congress theme was 'One World Many Voices' and my talk was enthusiastically received. The next day I left that unique city with my horizons raised. I was excited about finding new ways to support people all across the world to find their stammering voices at work.

There are 50 million people of employable age in the world who stammer. Millions of those voices remain silent today. Some are fearful of talking at work, many others are not even in work at all. We share a common bond. The opportunity for our generation is to enable many more of these 50 million stammering voices to be heard at work. Somebody supported us to find our full voice, and we can now help others to find theirs. Why wouldn't we?

50 million voices campaign

An international mindset towards stammering at work is now opening up. New collaborations are emerging between national support group leaders and with global employers and new allies.

In early 2019, I launched '50 Million Voices' in conjunction with enthusiastic leaders from the stammering communities in 13 countries across five continents: Australia, Canada, France, Germany, India, Ireland, Israel, Japan, Norway, Rwanda, South Africa, the United Kingdom and the United States. This international campaign aims to increase and accelerate change in the world of work for people who stammer. We're sharing and learning as we go.

Now only three months after its launch, 50 Million Voices has already started to stimulate positive change in several countries. Indeed, it's truly exciting to see how our team of talented leaders are creating paths forward to transform the world of work for the millions of people globally who stammer, every one of us with a unique voice – 50 million voices.

As they say in Japan, "Gambari Mashou!" – 'Let's go for it!'

"Even as the light fades quickly now,
You are not leaving,
You are arriving."

David Whyte

The man talks of 'leaving and arriving' as he tells people of his decision to withdraw from the EY partnership at December 2017. His friends tease him about retiring early and the firm present him with a lifetime impact award for his game-changing contribution to the disability and health agenda at EY.

He's leaving a leading global employer where embracing difference is now a value lived daily by its 250,000 partners and employees.

He's arriving in a new place where he will be able to give more time to changing the world of work for people who stammer. He's no longer one tentative voice. He's one amongst 50 million voices.

Acknowledgements

Many colleagues and allies have played valuable roles in the success of the EY Stammering Network (EYSN) and the ESN in so many different ways. In writing this chapter it has only been possible to name a small handful of them and therefore, in addition to those already mentioned, I'd particularly like to thank John Evans and Tim Fell, the former and current Chairs of the BSA, Steve Varley the Chair of EY in the UK and Ireland, Michelle Cuddihy, Dinesh Sathianathan and Chris Scott of the EYSN, and Carmen Savvas, my former executive assistant.

Thank you also to the Dominic Barker Trust for generously funding the independent evaluations of the ESN's workshops and pilot mentoring programme, as well as for their ever warm encouragement and advice.

Top tips: Sharing what's worked

We have made and walked our own path even though it has not always been a straight one! We are much clearer now about how to create a successful culture for people who stammer at work and how employers benefit from that too. Here are some top tips and ideas for others wishing to do the same:

- Remembering that our purpose is supporting people who stammer at work – the 1%.

- Aligning the stammering agenda with employers' own D&I agenda is critical – the 99%.

- Applying the principles of the social model of disability in tandem with D&I principles.

- Supporting Champions as leaders and role models in creating change in their own place of work.

- Collaborating with speech and language therapists in creating personal change.

- Attracting the right people with a passionate, caring and collaborative attitude.

- Living our shared values and keeping a sense of humour.

Over their eight years to date, the EYSN and the ESN have engaged in a wide range of activities:

For people who stammer:

- Support networks to connect and share
- 1-to-1 support and connections
- Various workshops
- Mentoring

For employers:

- Meetings about stammering, e.g., lunch & learn sessions
- Talks about stammering at work
- Educational workshops
- Best practice advice
- 'Understanding Stammering at Work' Guide

For everyone:

- Social events

- Themed events
- Fundraising activities
- ESN and employment component of BSA's website
- A voice in national and social media
- Speaking at meetings and conferences

References

Bailey, K., Harris, S.J., & Simpson, S. (2015). Stammering and the Social Model of Disability: Challenge and opportunity. *Procedia – Social and Behavioral Sciences, 193*, 13–24.

Butler, C. (2014). Wanted – straight talkers: Stammering and aesthetic labour. *Work Employment and Society, 28*(5), 718–734.

Employers Stammering Network and Employers Network for Equality & Inclusion. (2017, October). Understanding Stammering: A Guide for Employers. Retrieved February 12th, 2019, from https://www.stammering.org/help-information/topics/work/guide-employers-esn-and-enei

Gerlach, H., Totty, E., Subramanian, A., & Zebrowski, P. (2018). Stuttering and labor market outcomes in the United States. *Journal of Speech, Language, and Hearing Research, 61*(7), 1649–1663.

Speaking at the formal launch of the Defence Stammering Network, my maiden speech in the House of Lords no less.

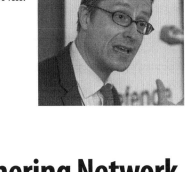

Fighting stigma against stammering: The Defence Stammering Network

Walter Scott

Long before co-founding the Defence Stammering Network, I felt a connection between stammering, the Armed Forces, and exclusion. Some 22 years earlier, aged 18, I had been rejected from the initial round of selection for the Army Scholarship scheme on the basis of my stammer; and a year later I was advised I would have little chance of success at getting a regular commission until I had addressed my 'speech problem'. Without speaking a word to anyone about this, that moment planted fears in my mind about future selection for any type of career. Although I recognized that Army service was not my natural calling, I had often day-dreamed of walking into Army headquarters and explaining why I thought its apparent attitude towards and handling of a potential officer with dysfluency was fundamentally wrong. In my late 20s, I joined the UK Ministry of Defence (MoD), the government department responsible for the British Armed Forces, mainly because I wanted to work with the Forces, but also because a little part of me wanted to complete some unfinished business.

Creation

I first met Jimmy Lang, then a sergeant-major in the British Army, at an evening event run by the British Stammering Association in early 2014. Jimmy had just spoken about his rise up the ranks whilst being a person who stammers. I liked how he chose to show his stammer: unabashed, with attitude, and even pride. That, I saw, was a quality with which I could do business. The Defence Stammering Network was conceived that evening. Jimmy and I had both read about another soldier called Emmanuel Ottih, who had started a stammering support group for soldiers based in Germany. We contacted Emmanuel and the three of us spent a month discussing what we could potentially do for stammering as an issue in relation to the Royal Navy, the Army, the Royal Air Force, MoD civil servants and Defence contractors. We had all had unfavourable experiences at points in our lives, and it was clear to us that the Armed Forces knew nothing of stammering. Four years later, the network has grown to over 100 members at all ranks and grades. As a team we have achieved more within and outside Defence than we could have ever imagined. So how has it happened?

Diverse team

We brought contrasting personal and career backgrounds to the network.

Jimmy had joined the Army from school. Despite a difficult start, he soon began to distinguish himself, climbing the ranks to Regimental Sergeant Major and later to Late Entry Officer while still relatively young. A natural military leader, he would identify a shared objective and then be unshakeable and methodical in completing it with as much energy and time as it required.

Emmanuel joined the Army's Logistics Corps as a non-commissioned officer relatively late, at 27. He had a degree in politics, but due to his stammer his fellow recruits assumed him unable to speak English. He described his early military life as 'difficult' and he was determined that no recruit should have the same experience as him. Brilliant at identifying niche opportunities, he had recently persuaded Forces TV to film him receiving speech therapy for a news feature, at the time a hugely courageous, unprecedented and impactful move.

I had entered the Civil Service with a degree, after some years of struggling with selection interviews. I had joined the Ministry of Defence as a corporate communications officer, and for 10 years had been working through a range of communication disciplines. I was inclined to lose focus, where Jimmy and Emmanuel would plough on, but I felt I could offer strength in presenting a case with nuances and build awareness and support.

So our combined backgrounds, styles of working and strengths created a wide pool of skills, knowledge and contacts, which widened as the network began to grow. We were well placed to influence military culture and the system, and to communicate our aims to a large and diverse audience. For all our differences, what we had in common were all the typical experiences, emotions and strengths that come with stammering.

Additionally, the fact that we were building a joint military-civilian network seemed to strike a chord at senior levels of Defence. While the Civil Service and Armed Forces operate in different legislative frameworks around disability issues, we were seeking to establish common ground and learning between the two sides, enforcing the point that no matter who you are, or where you work, a stammer presents common challenges.

Finding our purpose

It took us about a year to understand fully our objectives. In simple terms, we wanted to grow the network and provide mutual support, but how widely should we pitch it? And what else should we be trying to do? UK Defence is high-profile, complex, and globally influential in delivering a huge range of services involving the Armed Forces, civil servants, industry, and politicians, with perhaps a quarter of a million employees. What opportunities could this offer?

We agreed to spread our efforts across Defence as a whole, with the aim of supporting anyone, be they military, civilian, or contractor. We began by accumulating knowledge about what people who stammer are experiencing in the Defence system, from initial recruitment through their careers. This knowledge allowed us to create case studies, often inspiring examples, of people who stammer managing to do their jobs despite experiences of prejudice and discrimination. This could inspire while also helping to influence appropriate actions to improve policy and processes in the Armed Forces.

Another important objective became apparent when we received our first enquiry. It came from a military officer whose colleague was refused extra time for an oral assessment on a staff course. No one knew how to categorize her stammer in official disability terms. Not only did we have members who had encountered this before; we were also able to channel a professional view from the British Stammering Association to the officer, to remedy the problem. We realized that we were now empowered to provide advice and guidance on stammering, which until then had not been recognized in Defence as an issue.

As we started to receive more enquiries, we saw that in some instances we might need to go a step further than just guidance. When we received our first 'unfair treatment' case, from someone refused a place on a specialist training course due to his dysfluency, one of our officer members quickly contacted the relevant training establishment. She explained the nature of stammering, the decision was reversed, and the discrimination avoided.

It became increasingly clear to us just how low were levels of knowledge in Defence about stammering, from those managing equality & diversity and performance management policy, to those providing military medical support, reasonable adjustments, and recruiting. No one had ever asked for written policy, so the policy had never been written. The objective to educate and raise awareness was soon clear. Using media channels, and speaking or holding stalls at events and exhibitions, we started to disseminate key messages and information. In due course we developed some formal guidance that is now linked to written policy – a small but, for us, significant development. I realized that we were actually starting to change the culture around stammering in the Armed Forces.

Our profile grew not just internally to Defence, but outside it as well. While it was easy to assume that the Armed Forces was "No place for someone who stammers", here was a growing network of people who stammer who had been recruited to work for, and with, the Armed Forces. The fact that we existed – and were being encouraged to exist – as a staff network seemed to generate interest. When we eventually held our formal launch, the BBC and *Sunday Mail* were quick to request interviews.

Marketing for growth

Raising the profile of stammering can be a challenging task, and this network was never going to be an 'easy sell' in the military environment. Yet, clearing this hurdle, and marketing and publicizing the network was vitally important. As much as educating, we needed to cajole, inspire, and give confidence. We even needed to suggest that to not take interest presented a tacit risk.

The first basic challenge was keeping those who joined the network engaged and informed. We set up a presence on public-facing social media channels and an internal presence on the Defence intranet, allowing us to reach the Forces and Civil Service staff based all over the UK and the world, as well as the public. It was important that we created a sense of momentum to encourage those joining us, so we took it in turns to initiate conversation. This might involve reporting on an experience that day, providing a link to a media article, or asking advice. It all helped to create community value and drew out others' ideas and experiences.

We also made good use of the internal Defence communication channels, particularly the various internal magazines. In the first year, we tended to use our own individual stories – and simply our decision to team up – as the main hook. In time, this gave way to promoting our aims and successes, and other personal case studies. We would always reflect wider messages about stammering, such as the demographics, the neurological root cause, and our link to the UK Employers Stammering Network. Our stories and language were about people living and working with a stammer, as opposed to people 'conquering', 'beating' or 'overcoming' their dysfluency – which sends out the message that stammering itself is something that needs to be corrected.

With each intervention, more people joined us, each with their own story in response to what they had read. Our desire to speak out seemed to have an infectious edge. We were soon joined by a sergeant who had been decorated with a Mention in Despatches for his action in successfully evacuating a number of casualties during an intense combat situation in Afghanistan. During an hour under heavy fire from all directions, in between administering first aid, he had radioed extensive detailed instructions regarding each casualty to the Chinook base. And he had done so as someone with a lifelong stammer. He wrote a brilliant account of his experience, which generated public attention on Facebook.

After eight months, we had about 25 members – enough, we judged, for some TV coverage. Emmanuel made a pitch to Forces TV, and they proposed a documentary about our creation. I arranged for a reporter to interview six network members, along with the chief executive of the British Stammering Association, and the co-chair of the Employers Stammering Network. The finished 30-minute product, 'My War with Words', brilliantly portrayed the challenges and realities of military life with dysfluency and captured the value of supporting and understanding stammering for what it is. More than that, the reporter managed to show the value of camaraderie and the blossoming partnership between the Forces and the British Stammering Association. The documentary generated interest from many directions, including managers and unit commanders of people who stammer, and parents and guardians of young potential recruits, but also interest from members of the viewing public – and not just in the UK.

Three years later, we were contacted by the same reporter who wanted to relate the next chapter in our story. By now we had been joined by Brigadier James Woodham as our 'senior champion'. I organized for her to interview him and some other new network members, as well as Jimmy and myself. When 'Stammering: The Unspeakable Truth' hit the streets, the Forces TV press office secured appearances for Jimmy on BBC 5 Live and BBC Breakfast, and various 'back stories' about the making of the documentary; I was commissioned to write an article for the Forces TV website entitled 'My fight to remove the stammer stigma in the Armed Forces'.

Lucky timing

There is nothing unprecedented about people undertaking military service with a stammer. Yet what was perhaps unusual was the act of military personnel actively choosing to promote their stammering and doing so with pride. Ten years ago, they might have been penalized for cutting against the grain, yet now their stories were eagerly scooped up within the department as a learning opportunity. We were being encouraged to build a political force behind our neurological difference.

We were lucky in our timing, because this second decade of the 21st century has proven a rich time for progress with stammering awareness. The 2011 film 'The King's Speech' had sparked a media frenzy of interest in stammering. In 2013, Iain Wilkie, a senior partner at EY, and the then-shadow chancellor Ed Balls launched the Employers Stammering Network with the pioneering message that 'It is OK to stammer at work'. Added to that, it was now empirically recognized – at least in neuroscience circles – that stammering is rooted in neurological wiring, not personality, intellect, or confidence. The stigma of stammering was coming under fire from all sides.

Within Defence, circumstances favoured us with what appeared to be a concerted desire to get better at diversity & inclusion: recruiting from ethnic communities, intolerance of racism, homophobia and bullying, better awareness of mental health issues, and an uncomfortable sense of the low ratio of women on management boards and in senior management positions. There was recognition that changes to working culture would require staff to challenge the system, to offer up ideas and to innovate. Where Defence might have been traditionally seen as the preserve of white able-bodied males, there was now a recognition that a genuinely diverse and inclusive workforce was integral to operational delivery. And that meant readiness to learn and to improve at every turn.

From the moment that Emmanuel first approached British Forces Broadcasting, it was clear that we were unlocking genuine interest among colleagues in stammering. Our formal launch in July 2015 was supported by Mark Lancaster, MP, a Defence minister, and a number of senior officials. These included Sir Philip Rutnam, now Home Office permanent secretary and the Civil Service 'disability champion', who has continually supported our cause, and Lieutenant General Sir Andrew Gregory, the chief of military and civilian HR.

However, if the time was ripe for societal and workplace change, it was also clear that stammering support would not create its own momentum and moral arguments by itself. That was going to need forceful political will and encouragement – which would and could only come from among people who themselves stammer.

Collaboration

From the start we began building links with external organizations, including in the first instance the British Stammering Association, its Employers Stammering Network, and the City Lit stammering therapy team. This proved vital to ensuring the authenticity of what we were trying to do within Defence. It was often difficult to get people to understand that stammering was an issue worthy of consideration. Factors at play included low public awareness, scant media coverage, and the idea that 'the cause of stammering is not known'. This association with non-Defence organizations strengthened our official edge.

By forging a link with the Employers Stammering Network we were able to help its cause. We introduced the ESN to the director of Civil Service Diversity & Inclusion and soon we were asked to present a case for the whole UK Civil Service joining the ESN. After several meetings over the course of six months, the Civil Service membership was confirmed, representing a workforce of more than 400,000 people. It was an important moment which subsequently led to the creation of the Civil Service Stammering Network.

The public profile of the Defence Stammering Network has since opened a door to foreign collaboration. We were contacted via Facebook by a pilot officer of the US Coast Guard, asking for details of how and why we had set up as a group. His journey to securing a commission had been difficult and he was now inspired by the idea of a network to support and educate. We spoke via Skype for an hour one evening, and he went away to contact the US National Stuttering Association to see whether any other of its members were serving in the US Forces. A year later we were contacted by the new 'NSA Military Support' group, of which the pilot was one of the founding members. We are now in dialogue via social media and seeking projects on which the two networks can work together in the future.

Risk and courage

Over the last four years, I have identified and felt many reasons to give up the network. This was never a full-time vocation; it was only ever a voluntary activity. And given that many people who stammer experience rejection from employment opportunities due to their dysfluency at one stage or another – particularly on career paths that involve repeated competitive selection – to openly advertise myself as someone with dysfluent speech would likely have reduced my employability in some organizations. To some, it might look like I am an over-sensitive whinger, unable to cope with a few setbacks from a trivial condition. Of that I have been acutely aware. Added to which, there have been months when I wondered what the end-game was for the Defence Stammering Network – in practical terms, human beings being a tribal species, what could we actually hope to change in terms of stigma?

What has kept me going on this journey has been the camaraderie of Jimmy and Emmanuel – the original commitment that we made to being successful in a Sandhurst carpark one afternoon – and the subsequent camaraderie of those who have joined us in a steady trickle over the years. Each new joiner, each with their own story, every case where we have intervened, has added to the argument for continuing. What has also kept me going has been the interest of so many different people and organizations, and a sense that we are having an impact on attitudes. But to continue having an impact, we have to keep the entity alive. Without it, the default view of stammering – as a trivial, slightly off-putting nervous character trait – would soon reassert itself over the precious inches of territory we have gained.

Our official launch in July 2015 in the House of Lords gave us a very clear indication that we were heading in the right direction and it was followed by a series of invitations to speak at equality & diversity and health fairs in different parts of Defence. In political terms, we appeared to have hit the zeitgeist, and that was both exhilarating and cathartic. At the 200-strong Royal Navy diversity & inclusion conference, I decided to share my rejection from Army Scholarship selection 24 years before, and told them the story of the sergeant who won a Mention in Despatches, ending with an impassioned question:

"What are these jobs that people who stammer cannot do? I want to know what they are."

But what if all this should jeopardize future career avenues for me personally? To my mind, you can invest your energy in securing the best financial and formal status arrangements for yourself. Or you can focus your energy in the wider circumstances for the society in which you live. A tiny minority manage both, but for me I know that I could not possibly work for an employer or a cause which is not fully accepting of my way of speaking, or my urge to campaign for wider awareness and acceptance.

Looking forward

The Defence Stammering Network now has more than 100 members. Some are proactive in raising local awareness, distributing DSN literature, and briefing colleagues. The majority are happy just to participate in online conversations, to observe and be kept informed. As stammering can be highly isolating when hidden, there is value and security simply in belonging to a kindred group with a collective interest. It is now clear that unfair treatment towards anyone who stammers in Defence is likely to be followed up.

A few of our members have received formal recognition for this work. In the Queen's Birthday Honours 2016, Jimmy was made a Member of the British Empire (MBE), with a citation that read:

> "...his passionate efforts and success in supporting those who stammer reinforces the inherent goodness of the man."

It was a well-earned decoration because Jimmy had worked harder than anyone to promote stammering as an issue for the Forces. Emmanuel was also honoured with an MBE the following year. That gave me a huge ego boost.

On a personal level I do still harbour concerns about societal attitudes. Despite what the Equality Act provides for, if someone finds the sight or sound of dysfluent speech embarrassing or even insulting, or if a profession places higher value in blemish-free speech, then individuals are more likely to act prohibitively in the workplace, albeit through subtle means. It astonishes – and frankly infuriates – me that while speech is so vital to wellbeing, society remains so poorly informed about stammering. After centuries of muddled, misinformed understanding about the causes, discrimination and bullying, there is much more work to be done on building greater acceptance and understanding. Yet, I believe that in the UK we are making early progress at dismantling this ancient prejudice.

I am particularly proud of the stance I have taken with Jimmy and Emmanuel, supported by the British Stammering Association and many others, in beginning to change attitudes. I am excited by the work that lies ahead.

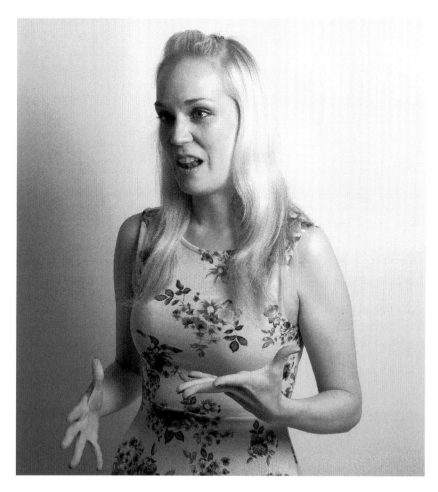

Picture 1: Satu Tuulia Nygren

Capturing the stammering aesthetic

A project by Alda Villiljós , Sigríður Fossberg Thorlacius, Sveinn Snær Kristjánsson and Málbjörg (the National Stuttering Association in Iceland) to document the movements and tics of people who stammer and, more importantly, to celebrate them as something unique and personal.

'The stammering aesthetic is an aspect of the person you may often witness when you meet them face to face, but one which is never shown on a still photograph. And yet, it is often an important aspect of their identity.'

Reprinted gratefully with permission from Sveinn Snær Kristjánsson and those pictured.

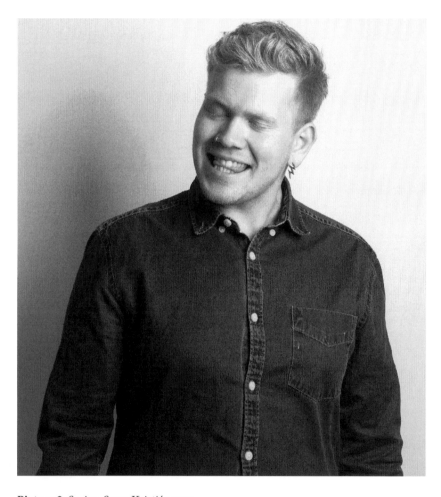

Picture 2: Sveinn Snær Kristjánsson

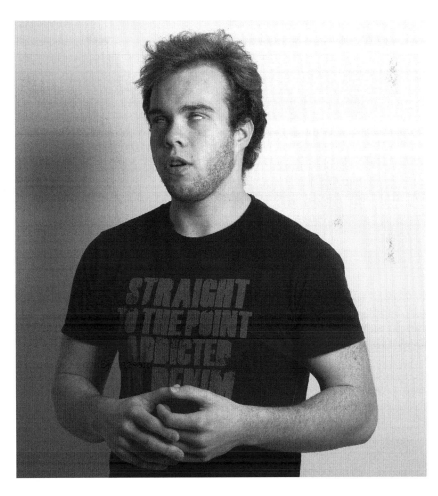

Picture 3: Andri Bjarnason

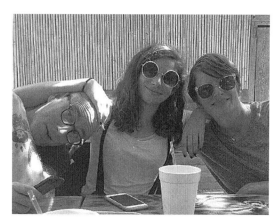

I hate that there is a big styrofoam cup in the photo,
but I love it anyway!

A journey in eight events

Elizabeth Wislar

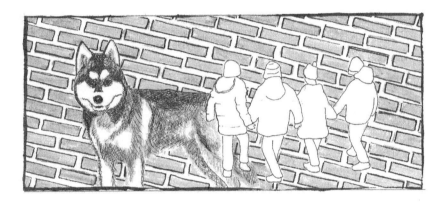

1 Ignorance

"Why does she talk like that?"

It was Paul who asked. The same Paul who threw up all over his desk at our Valentine's Day party last year in 1st grade. Paul who always wore brown corduroy pants, even in the summer.

He tugged at my mom's arm trying to get her attention. "Hey, why does she talk that way?"

My mom was there at my school for show and tell. My classmates were all huddled around us wearing their winter coats and mittens. She'd brought two of our huskies, Jack and Misty, and we were showing my class how we hook them up to a toboggan to race. I had been in the middle of proudly showing my class how I brushed my dogs. Everyone wanted a tuft of fur.

"Why does she talk funny?" he asked again.

I pretended I didn't hear him and kept brushing Jack who was smiling from all the attention. Did I talk funny? I was starting to think I did. Some older girls on my school bus had been asking me weird questions and laughing at my answers. My brother told the bus driver and they got moved.

I looked at my mom to see what she would say to Paul, mostly because I wanted to know what he meant. But my mom didn't say anything and looked embarrassed like when my brother blew his nose in his sleeve in the checkout line at the Piggly Wiggly. She looked at Paul with her mouth open a little bit like she was about to say something.

"Go stand by the wall," my teacher, Miss White, hissed at him. He was in trouble for asking.

I looked at my mom. Did I talk funny? Now I was afraid to ask.

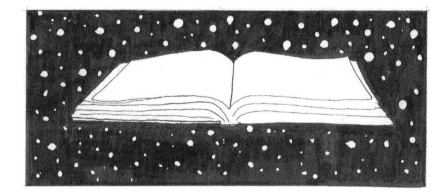

2 Loathing

I could feel a drip of sweat trickling down my side as I counted the kids ahead of me again. Four until it was my turn. I looked at the paragraphs again too, hoping I had counted wrong. The one I would have to read was long and had words like Michelangelo and Renaissance. I'd never get through those words. I would have to do what I always did and pretend I couldn't read them.

On the first day of school, my mom had told my teacher, Mr Z, I stuttered. He wasn't supposed to make me read out loud in class if I didn't want to. Maybe he forgot, or didn't believe her. Now it was like he was trying to make me prove it.

I muddled through my turn, quietly reading out the words I knew I could say easily and letting my classmates impudently read the ones I couldn't. It was even more humiliating because some of the words I couldn't say were easy, but I was determined to not let the kids at this new school hear me stutter.

At my old school I was teased a lot, even by my friends. Kids made fun of the way I said my name, or they'd snicker if I stuttered on an answer. But they knew me; they'd heard me talk since first grade. Here the kids didn't know a thing about me. They all seemed so perfect and gifted. I didn't trust them at all.

So I was doing everything I could think of not to stutter here. It was obvious no one liked me, so at recess I just sat on the bench and read. In class, if I got asked a question, I would just shrug. It seemed better for everyone to think I didn't know the answers than to stutter on them. Even when it was time for me to go to speech therapy on Tuesday and Thursday afternoons, and the kids would say, "It's time for your special ed class," I didn't care.

In speech I learned ways to not stutter, like starting out really soft and slow. I was really good when I was in the therapy room, but as soon as I left, it seemed like the tricks I learned didn't work. My mom and stepfather told me I wasn't trying hard enough. They called me lazy. I learned really fast how to stop using words I knew I'd stutter on. This made my mom and stepfather think I was using my speech tricks. If I went through a whole dinner without stuttering, my mom would even give me extra dessert.

Not using words I'd stutter on was working in school too. I'd gotten through most of the fall this way. Except one day just after winter break, a blizzard hit and we had to stay in the classroom for recess. I had just started reading a book I'd gotten for Christmas: *Island of the Blue Dolphins*, by Scott O'Dell. I was absorbed in the warmth of the beach. I didn't hear Mr Z come up behind me, but suddenly he snatched the book out of my hand and told me harshly that I "couldn't possibly be reading that book". I tried to get it back, but he held it out of my reach. He'd said, "if you can read this, then read me the first page out loud."

I tried. I tried to use the things I was practising in speech therapy: starting slow and breathing out with my words. Like always, it didn't work and I got stuck on the third word. Nothing would come out.

"I didn't think so." He threw the book back on my desk and walked away.

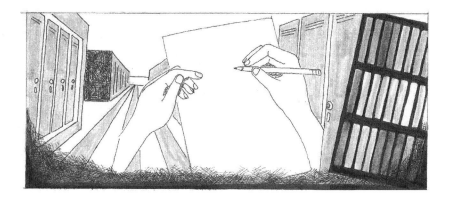

3 Isolation

The chalk dust on my fingers was giving my sandwich a bruised look, but I didn't want to go to the girl's room to wash my hands. I'd have to walk past the others and I didn't want to draw attention to myself. I turned up the volume on my walkman and ground the chalky pastel into my drawing. It was all I could do to keep from scrawling the word 'betrayal' across the still life.

It had been Ms Pulaski's idea at first – me coming to her classroom for lunch. Earlier in the year she'd found me in the clinic next to the teacher's lounge. The nurse wasn't there so I was just sitting by the door with my head in my hands. I was sweaty and couldn't breathe, my heart alternately leaping and stopping for what seemed like minutes at a time. I thought I was dying.

She must have recognized the symptoms because she had helped me take deep breaths as she counted backward from 10 slowly. She explained what a panic attack was and asked if I had one before. I nodded. I had them all the time.

She'd walked me slowly back to her classroom at the end of the Freshman hall – a room I knew well since I was taking all the art classes the school would allow. She'd microwaved me a cup of chamomile tea and let me sit there quietly through the lunch break.

Then it just became what I did. As soon as the bell rang for lunch and everyone made their way to the cafeteria, I walked against the current to her classroom. Sometimes we'd just work on our own projects and eat quietly listening to James Taylor and Cat Stevens, but sometimes we'd talk. She'd tell me about her cat or her cantankerous nephew, Evan. Sometimes she'd ask me questions: what did I want to do after high school or what art schools was I applying to? Like always, I tried to concoct sentences without words I'd stutter on. I talked around subjects and often left out important details. Sometimes though, my stutter would sneak up on me and slip out. It would appear as a hard and ugly block that I felt would never end. My face burned red, but Ms Pulaski never acted surprised or alarmed. She'd just keep talking like nothing had happened.

Months went by and the art room became my refuge. It felt safer than my own home where my speech was always under inspection. Going there for lunch was my favourite part of the day.

I don't know why Ms Pulaski invited the other kids. Maybe she thought I needed to make friends or maybe she thought her room could be a safe place for other lost kids. Whatever the reason, I was terribly hurt.

I listened to their conversation – the way their words came so easily. I would never be able to talk to them. I would need to find a new place to go.

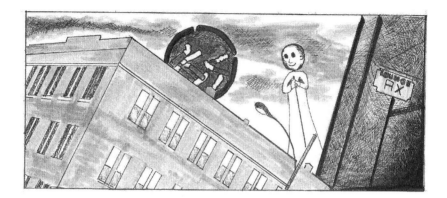

4 Deception

"Have you read any Grace Paley?" I shouted into Dan's ear.

"What?"

I pushed away his stringy hair. "Have you read anything by Grace Paley?"

"No. Should I?"

"I just started a book of short stories and I really love it."

"I can't really hear you. Do you want to go outside?"

"No!" Despite the heat and the sticky bodies pressed close around us, this was the perfect environment for me to talk. I could barely hear myself, but I could tell by the lack of tension in my throat and mouth that I wasn't going to stutter.

It had been during a Tortoise show at Lounge Ax the previous year that I realized I could speak without stuttering if there was a loud band playing. It worked in other loud situations as well, like when the 'L' train was pulling up to the platform or on a plane that was taking off. I tried to take advantage of these situations whenever I could.

My collection of tricks to not stutter was getting larger and more versatile. Most of the people I'd met since moving to Chicago didn't even know that I had a stutter. I'd even recently taken up smoking. If I started to get stuck on a word, I'd just take a drag off my cigarette, and no one knew. Sometimes I would speak with an accent that morphed from Irish to Russian to sort of Scandinavian. Chicago was full of accents and I rarely got called out on it. No one had any clue.

When I really had to talk and there wasn't loud music, and an accent wouldn't work, I eased into my words using other sounds or words.

"Yeeeeaaaaahhhaaaaahhhhbagle," I'd tell the food prepper at my job. I worked in a coffee shop where it was completely acceptable to take someone's order without talking to them.

I knew I came across as quirky, but everyone I knew was quirky. It wasn't unusual to see someone at a party wearing a paper Halloween costume, or walking a pot-bellied pig down the street. My neighbourhood of Wicker Park was filled with artists, musicians, actors, writers and everyone was fairly accepting of each other's eccentricities – everyone was putting on a show. We were all escaping our old uncomfortable lives and terrible childhoods. We were all burning bridges and creating new identities. My friend Jenny was fond of saying that no person worth knowing had had an easy time when they were young.

I was living in one big piece of performance art along with everyone else and it was perfect, because in this performance, I no longer stuttered.

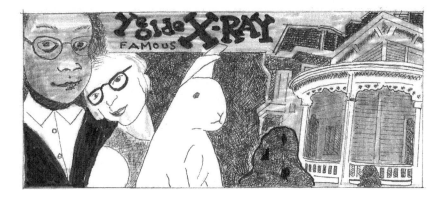

5 Denial

It took me weeks to finally send them a message. I'd scoured their Church of Craft MySpace page dozens of times. They seemed so nice and cool and the idea of a group of people meeting to do crafts was appealing; just the type of thing I was looking for.

After getting my teaching degree, my husband, daughter and I had moved out of Chicago to a sleepy college town in the southeastern part of the country. I was struggling to find a niche. I felt a void when it came to art and music. These had been so important to me in the city.

I thought of stuttering as a problem I used to have. Even though I was aware of my speech all the time, I didn't face many of the blocks and repetitions I had in my younger years. Sure I still had to change words sometimes – a lot of times maybe, but didn't most people?

It seemed soon after we moved like we were going to become friends with a couple. I worked with the wife and they had invited us to their home for dinner. We'd sat on their large front porch trying to find something in common between our northern and southern pasts. It had been painfully awkward and I had stuttered more than in years. In the weeks after the dinner, I let the potential friendship dissolve out of embarrassment and adopted the persona of an introvert recovering from city life. I just wanted to spend time with my husband and daughter.

But now I was looking to find my niche and people like I used to know back in Chicago. My heart pounded as I walked from my car to the storefront called X-Ray Cafe where the Church of Craft meeting was being held. I'd decided to walk past once and see if it looked safe. I was so relieved to see only a few people in the storefront. They were sitting on the floor with sheets of colourful felt laid out before them. They welcomed me by name with accents I recognized as northern. I was so relieved.

I joined them on the floor, nervously opened my wicker sewing basket and took out the stuffed rabbit I was working on. I had based it on an antique silk rabbit I'd found at a little shop in Savannah. It was a hit.

I hadn't anticipated how much talking I was going to have to do. The leaders of the group, Missy and Raoul, took turns asking me questions about Chicago, my family and what had brought us to Athens. I tried to answer them carefully and accurately using safe, brief answers. It took everything I had; it had been a long time since I'd spoken with strangers.

On the drive home I reviewed everything I had said, relieved I hadn't stuttered at all. That was still the most important thing.

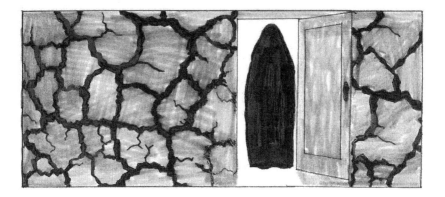

6 Revelation

We'd been circling the same area for close to an hour with the overwhelming Barcelona street map folded to just show the area around the hotel. The neighbourhood was a mass of one-way streets and multilaned roundabouts. Cars, taxis and scooters whizzed past our rental car. It was a nightmare. The hotel seemed to be on a one-way street that had no access. How could that be?

We finally made a plan: my husband would pull up next to a taxi and I'd jump out and ask the driver how to reach the hotel. This was a great plan, except for one thing: I could not switch words in Spanish.

"¿...D d d d d dónde es es es es está este hhhhhhotel?" I pointed to the address on the hotel registration form, hoping my stutter came across as uncertainty about the language.

The taxi driver laughed and pointed to the end of the street explaining that we had to drive across a square to reach our hotel entrance.

This situation had worked out okay, but it was situations like this that made me feel like I had no control. It was times like this where my veil of fluency was challenged the most.

Control was the way I coped. I kept everything under control. My house, car and classroom were always tidy. I woke at the same time, ate the same breakfast and drove the same way to work every day. Even then there were unpredictable events that happened.

I could count times I'd completely lost control and most were not as funny as the time in Barcelona. I'd developed a blood clot after the birth of my daughter. There was the time my dad had hit his head and wasn't making sense and the time I totalled my car. Events like these challenged the tight control I kept over my speech. They created situations where avoiding certain words was impossible.

I'd never felt the loss of control as much as when my mother fell ill from a complication after knee surgery. Starting from the night I had to call an ambulance to meeting with her priest to plan a funeral, I had to speak with so many people, all the while dealing with my own fear and grief. For more than a month from the time my mother fell ill to when she finally passed away, my sense of control crumbled. My anxiety peaked. I struggled with my speech more than I had in years. It became much harder to think of myself as fluent anymore.

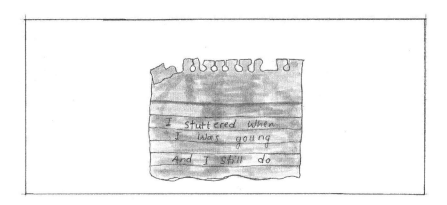

7 Acceptance

There she was at my classroom door. I had asked her to come by and talk and now she was there waiting for an explanation. Her face was a mix of concern and curiosity and I couldn't blame her.

From that first faculty meeting years before, when she'd introduced herself as a new teacher and a person who stuttered, I had avoided her. If she came in the teacher's lounge, I'd leave. If she sat near me in a meeting, I'd make an excuse to move. It was ridiculous but I didn't want to hear her stutter or, worse yet, what if she could hear it in me?

But now we were working on the same hall, with the same grade level. We had planning meetings together. I could no longer avoid her. She would eventually figure it out. I had known for a while that I needed to start coming clean about my speech. The control I'd worked on for my whole life had begun to crumble and I was unable to count on my tricks working. I knew eventually she would hear it and wonder why I never told her or, worse yet, think that I was mocking her.

I invited her in and asked her to sit. I kept the fluorescent lights turned off. Maybe it would be easier to talk in the dark.

"So, um…" I couldn't think of the words to use. There would be no way to switch words this time. I always stuttered on the word 'stutter.' And the years I spent keeping this secret made it so hard to dig up and spill out.

"Um," I took a few deep breaths.

"I feel like I should be worried." She got up and came over to sit closer to me. She was scared she had done something. I could tell.

"No! No! It's me." I felt the burning sensation of a cry starting in my throat.

"I need to…" I made a writing motion with my hand and grabbed a pen and notepad from my desk.

"Okay?" She was obviously very confused by my actions.

The note wasn't the solution I was hoping for. I couldn't decide what exactly to write on that either. I finally wrote *I stuttered when I was young.* But I knew I had to go farther so I added, *and I still do.*

I handed her the note and resisted the urge to cover up my face. Tears rolled down my cheeks and my shoulders started to shake.

"Oh my God, I had no idea!"

There was so much now that I wanted to tell her.

We hugged and sat together for a very long time. We talked about how hard it was when we were kids and how we dealt with events in our lives now. I had never talked to another person who stuttered about stuttering before. I had no idea how empowering and cathartic it could be.

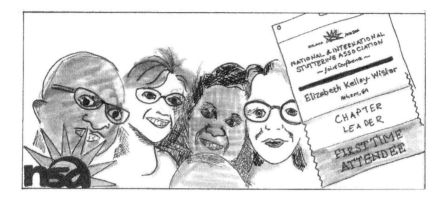

8 Gain

I have never been one for taking risks. Going to the NSA/IFA World congress in Atlanta was one of the biggest risks I'd ever taken. I was profoundly nervous.

Fortunately, I'd made a friend through StutterSocial, Carl, who was just as nervous as I was. I met him and his roommate in the lobby on the first morning and after a hug, the three of us decided to go look for coffee and breakfast. We walked around the hotel lobby and then outside. Listening to them speak and stutter while walking down a busy street was weird.

We went to Starbucks for coffee and I stuttered. I fought the urge to change my order from large latte and cinnamon scone to something easier, but I didn't. I had my friends with me.

As we went to workshops and hung out my circle of friends constantly grew. I saw other people from StutterSocial friends and introductions were made. I even reached a point where I could walk up to someone and introduce myself. I had never in my life been in a room with more than one other person who stuttered. Going to the NSA conference gave me the opportunity to be in rooms with hundreds of others who shared many of the same experience I had.

While community and friendship has been the biggest gain from finally owning that I am a person who stutters, there have been so many others. It has opened up a new connection with my students at work. For years I have worked with students with disabilities but never admitted that I too was disabled. Gaining this perspective has allowed me to connect with them and see similar obstacles in their lives. I have also found more direction in my creativity through writing and art. There is so much pain and ugliness in those years I spent loathing and hiding the way I talked. I hope to dig it up and reform it into something useful and perhaps even beautiful. Lastly, I have even developed a sense of leadership I once thought was unattainable or undesirable. Being an NSA chapter leader has given me an opportunity to reach out to others who might be in the place where I was years ago and to help them find their voices.

It's truly ironic to think about how something I spent so much of my life avoiding and refusing to acknowledge has now become my sense of purpose. I know my journey has not ended and I am eager to see where it will take me next.

It's complicated: CP and stuttering

Kristel Kubart

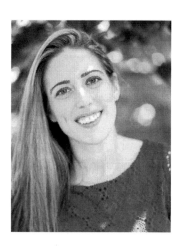

Growing up with cerebral palsy and with stuttering, I got a lot of unwanted attention. People weren't quite sure of what to make of the way that I walked or talked. I often felt like people were watching me, trying to figure me out. It's not every day you see a skinny little blonde girl walking on her tiptoes with her left foot turned in. Neither is it all that common to see that same girl completely blocking on her name, face all twisted and no sound coming out. They didn't know what to think or how to respond. Sometimes they would stare, or laugh, or do a double take. Oftentimes, they still do.

Coming to accept and eventually take pride in my disabilities has been a long, tough journey. There is so much pressure to conform to the norm. Over the years, with help from loving and supportive people, and some hard work on my part, I've grown more comfortable with my own voice and my own body. I wish that I could say that I have equal amounts of acceptance for both of my disabilities, but if I'm being honest it has been a struggle for me. I feel differently about each. My difficulty with accepting both of my disabilities to the fullest likely stems from the way society handles people who are different and how I have internalized those messages.

People are often given the message that being disabled inherently makes them 'less than'. As such, my goal growing up was to seem as able-bodied as possible, despite all of the physical and emotional pain that it caused. I wanted nothing more than to 'fit' into the able-bodied world. Over time, I've learned the importance of embracing my differences, to let my disabilities be seen, and to advocate for my needs. I've learned that I can have a very lovely life as a disabled person, filled with community and unique experiences. The challenges I face as I learn how to be my authentic self have given me a deeper understanding of who I am. These experiences have also helped me to empathize with others who face similar challenges.

Cerebral palsy: Different but whole

I'm grateful for the fact that, when I was a child, I had opportunities to speak openly about my cerebral palsy (CP). From my parents, I got the message that it was okay for me to do physical activities in my own way. I had a very happy childhood. My mom tells stories of watching me running on the sidewalk outside our suburban Long Island home. I would fall, hop back up, and then immediately go back to running. It wouldn't be long before I would fall again, but it didn't bother me. I have scars on my knees, but also wonderful memories of evenings spent playing outdoor games with my brother Tim and our friends from the neighbourhood. I ran with a gait that was lopsided and laboured, but when I ran, I was smiling.

My parents never wanted my CP to put limits on the experiences I could have. They gave me lots of opportunities to enjoy being in my body. I felt like they encouraged me to do what other kids were doing. Sometimes they even made modifications for me without my realizing it. I would tell people that I loved to hike and had no idea that when my family went hiking, my parents would turn us around and head back after we were only a short way into the trail, so it wouldn't be too strenuous for me.

Although my parents tried to shield me from feeling disabled, my cerebral palsy made me stand out. Consequently, I had to learn that it was OK to be myself and do things in my own unique way. I was not able to hide the fact that I walked differently because it was immediately obvious to others. As a child, if my unique walk wasn't enough to turn heads, I also wore thick braces on my legs that went up to my knees. Even though they were helping me walk, they were also clunky, impinging and foreign. They made me feel self-conscious and I got lots of curious looks and stares wherever I went. I hated being stared at for my CP, and I still do. In society disabilities aren't normalized enough so people tend to stare. I learned that stares will undoubtedly happen, the only thing I can control is how I feel about those stares. I've had to learn to think differently about the unwanted attention, and it's not always easy.

In addition to my parents, my physical therapist, Bonnie, was another person who offered guidance and encouragement. Bonnie spoke more directly to me than my parents did about CP and its impact on me. Over time, I learned that CP is something I would have my whole life. When I went to physical therapy I was able to work on it without feeling the pressure of having to get rid of it or feeling like I failed when I continued to be affected by it. When Bonnie led me through strengthening exercises, she would be right next to me on the floor or cheering me on as I stepped forward on a balance beam. Rather than feeling isolated by my disability, I felt very close to her, seen, and understood.

Going to physical therapy was also time I got to share with my mom. The drive to Bonnie's office was a ritual we shared each week on Wednesdays and Saturdays. My mother was afraid to say the words 'cerebral palsy' to me. She didn't want to give it a name, but Bonnie told her that I would hear it from someone at some point. She suggested it would be best if I heard it from my parents. For my mother, the name was frightening. She thought it might upset me. For my mom, it carried images of pain and struggle, but for me, it was just a label to describe my experience. When I was 6 years old she faced the moment she had dreaded and told me I had cerebral palsy. I didn't get upset, and I went right back to playing.

Stuttering: Shame and silence

With regards to my stutter, many people, even those I was very close to, were reticent to talk about it or even acknowledge it. That silence was, in many ways, more painful than people's stares or laughter. It made me feel like stuttering was something that should be hidden. At this point in my life, I try to foster open conversations about stuttering, cerebral palsy, and other disabilities. Breaking that silence is an important way to help people realize that being different doesn't have to be a bad thing.

For my CP I had a team of people who were there for me, supporting me, and on my side. The same couldn't be said about my stuttering. Conversations about how I felt about my stutter were few and far between. I don't have any memories of my parents sitting me down and telling me that I had a stutter. Even when I would struggle desperately to get a word out, my dad might say something like, "Oh don't you hate it when you get stuck like that", but we didn't really talk about it much beyond that. I really wanted to say words fluently, and when I wasn't able to I felt extremely embarrassed and ashamed. At the time I wished I could figure out a way to speak without a stutter, which I tried desperately to do.

There's a genetic component to stuttering and it often runs in families. My dad stutters too, and when he was young he was bullied for the way he spoke. His response was to make the bullies laugh. His strategy to deal with his stuttering has always been to be extremely outgoing and funny. When I was growing up he tried to model that for me. He told stories all the time, and loved being the centre of attention. As a child, this was something I was convinced I couldn't do. I was extremely embarrassed every time I stuttered and I could not bear the shame of it. I tried very hard to say words fluently, which made me get stuck on them even more. I didn't know letting myself stutter on words freely would help the words come out. So for the most part I chose to not say much of anything. Not speaking was my coping strategy. To avoid the pain of embarrassment, I chose silence, which caused its own deep pain.

School: Learning to hide

In my experience children become more aware of their differences as they get older. That was definitely true for me. Third grade was the last year I remember being able to speak in front of a crowd without fear. I was stuttering then, but I wasn't bothered by it. That year, I read the book *If You Give A Mouse A Cookie* in front of my class for show and tell. I'm sure I stuttered as I read, but I don't remember getting stuck or feeling afraid or embarrassed as I spoke in front of all the other children.

Soon after, that changed. In fourth grade, I remember my teacher would go around the room and have each child take a turn reading a paragraph out loud. This frightened me to death. I was very afraid that I would be judged and that my classmates would laugh at me. I was ashamed that I couldn't even finish a sentence without getting stuck. I knew what the words were, I just couldn't voice them. Even as I write this paragraph, the pain I felt as a child comes rushing back to me. It's a pain that's very hard to put into words. I was so embarrassed that I started anticipating when my turn would come and asking to go to the bathroom to avoid it. On a day when I was supposed to give a presentation, I would pretend to be sick so I could stay home from school. I felt like hiding was the only way to protect myself.

Unlike CP, I felt I might be able to hide my stutter. The belief that it could be hidden held me back. I suffered with my stuttering alone. I never went to speech therapy. I didn't make it known how much it was impacting me emotionally and practically in my daily life. No one knew that I was constantly thinking about it and trying to avoid it. Since CP is impossible to hide, some might think it harder to deal with than stuttering; however, its conspicuousness actually helped me to face it.

Looking back on that time in my life I realize I would have benefitted from a speech therapist who understood the nuances of stuttering and normalized my experiences with it. But my father was sceptical whenever the possibility of speech therapy was raised. When he was in his own speech therapy as a child, the only focus was on teaching fluency strategies. Those strategies didn't work for him, and that led him to think that speech therapy wasn't useful.

His experience is a common one. Many speech therapists don't focus at all on one's thoughts and feelings about stuttering. They usually push fluency strategies instead of understanding and self-acceptance which is the most important thing. Without good speech therapy, I felt that my stuttering was too overwhelming, a burden I could not carry.

College: Fear and avoidance

College was a low point for me in dealing with my stutter. It was the time in my life when I was most self-conscious and I struggled greatly. Meeting new people was scary since I stuttered severely when saying my name. If I couldn't say 'Kristel' fluently, I avoided introducing myself all together. In my junior year, I was a manager for the men's basketball team, a group of people who enjoyed god-like status on our campus. Somehow, I served for an entire season without ever telling any of the players my name. They eventually learned my name, but it was still really painful for me. I avoided many social interactions while in college. Making new friends became more difficult. Friendships are formed as people share stories with one another, and telling stories was almost impossible for me.

In my classes, I would beg any professor who assigned a presentation to let me write an extra paper instead. In a philosophy class sophomore year, each student was given a turn to give a two-minute explanation of the assigned reading. I wrote out everything I wanted to say. Alone in my dorm room, I practised again and again, but when the moment arrived, I couldn't get through it. Every word was a struggle. I had friends in the class. They never mentioned what happened. I felt disgusted with myself and I was convinced the class felt the same way. I wanted to pretend like this never happened. I thought I pushed this memory into a corner, but I still can connect to how unbelievably painful it was.

Senior year, while studying in the common area of my dorm, I managed to get through a conversation with a guy without stuttering. He was handsome, and I really liked him. When he asked me out, I was elated. We went to lunch at Crossroads, the fast food joint on campus, but sitting next to him I could barely talk at all. I had so much to say, but my fear of stuttering got in the way. There wasn't a second date. I always dreamed of having a boyfriend, but I was convinced that my stuttering would make it impossible. My speech made me feel like I didn't deserve love and I was unworthy of the attention.

Growth and acceptance

I hit a turning point with my stuttering a year after college. I found out about a stuttering support group near my parents' house and I decided to attend. It was in the days before GPS and I remember I was trying to find my way in the dark. I got very lost, but eventually I got there. When I arrived, I met Lee, a speech therapist whose son stutters. Lee was upset that no one else attended the support group that night. I, however, was grateful that I had an opportunity to talk with her one-on-one. She believes passionately that someone who stutters should never feel ashamed of it.

In that moment, I decided that I wanted to be a speech therapist too. When I told this to Lee, she was excited, but pointed out that I had never had good speech therapy. I asked her when we should start. This time, the goal wasn't fluency. Instead, it was about self-acceptance and changing how I manage my own stuttering. Lee was the first person to say to me that it was OK to stutter. When she said it, it resonated with me. I'm not sure if I would have been as open to it at a younger age, but at this point in my life, I was ready to take in that message.

My path to acceptance started with becoming more desensitized to my stuttering. In the past, when I stuttered on a word, I would push through it with a lot of tension. I would feel extremely embarrassed and want to run away. With Lee, instead of running away, I would stay in the stutter. I learned that I could be in the moment of stuttering without freaking out. Lee challenged me to let the stuttering happen. As I stopped fighting it, I could stutter with less tension and struggle.

Part of the way that I became desensitized to stuttering was through voluntary stuttering, or stuttering on purpose. When I stuttered on purpose, I was doing the thing that I was always so fearful and ashamed of, but I was doing it on my own terms. For me, stuttering on purpose made it easier to keep eye contact while stuttering. Before speech therapy, I would always look away when I stuttered, and I would assume that my listener was as uncomfortable as I was. As I challenged myself to voluntary stutter and maintain eye contact, I realized that the more comfortable I was with my stuttering, the more comfortable my listener would be.

Shortly after I met Lee, she told me about an organization she founded called FRIENDS, which focuses on empowering young people who stutter and their families. I found out they were having a one-day workshop in St. Louis. Although it was impulsive, I bought a plane ticket from my home in New York a day before the workshop was to begin. I remember thinking that I had to be there. It ended up being one of the best decisions I have ever made. At that workshop, I heard people speak openly about their experiences of stuttering. I found great comfort discovering an environment where few people acted like their stutter was something they had to hide.

After that, I started to meet many other adults who stutter that I admire. People that I came to realize are strong, beautiful, and brave. They were doing things in the world that matter while stuttering. I'm grateful every day for those relationships. Meeting these people allowed me to develop a sense of pride in stuttering while being a part of this amazing community. The experience of talking about stuttering in speech therapy and with other people who stutter helped me get to a place where stuttering no longer felt like a burden. Instead, it felt like a part of my identity I was happy to embrace.

The excitement I felt when I started to see my stuttering in a new way never faded. I began to consider the possibility that I could assist others in changing the way that they view their stuttering too. It's now been almost 10 years that I have been a speech therapist and I love it. It is something that I was meant to do. I am both passionate and committed to conveying the message that it's OK to stutter. My experience of my disabilities has shaped the way I practise with my clients. I have empathy for their struggle and a belief that they can relate to their stuttering in a new way. As a speech therapist, I offer my clients an opportunity to speak openly about their experiences with their stutter – the difficulties, fears, embarrassments, opportunities, and joys it often brings. There is so much beauty that can happen when my clients create a disability-friendly environment, rather than try to conform to an able-bodied world.

Pride and advocacy

Having pride in my disabilities means being able to talk about them openly. I have come to realize that to expect people to ask questions about my disabilities goes against what they have been taught. People think that asking about the way I move or the way I speak is rude. The silence that made me feel like my stutter was something I should hide came from people's efforts to be polite. Now I have realized I can create opportunities to talk about my experiences, and when I do, it helps to de-stigmatize topics related to disability. I enjoy having open conversations with people, and I think these kinds of discussions can accumulate into larger societal change.

As I have become more engaged in advocacy related to stuttering, I have started to think about how I can be even more accepting and open about my CP. When I was younger it was my stuttering that was hard to accept, now as an adult it's the opposite. There are times when I find it difficult to ask for help, even when I know I need it. This past year I started using a wheelchair when I go to the airport. I struggle with walking up and down stairs. When I have to cross a street in icy weather, I have to ask a stranger to let me hold their arm for support so I don't fall. I usually feel embarrassed to ask, even though people tell me they are happy I did.

At this point in my life, I am thinking more seriously than ever about the damage I sometimes do to my body when I push myself harder than I should. As I get older I'm finding that I have to modify the way that I do things even more than I used to. Each additional modification takes me one step further from the 'norm'. I know that I need to embrace each change and accept it as just the way I do things. Sometimes this comes easily and other times not so much. I am taking more pride in these things that are making me increasingly more different than the able-bodied.

My husband Jason has been an important companion on my journey to combat societal stigma of disability. As an able-bodied person who doesn't stutter he has always encouraged me to view my disabilities as a beautiful part of who I am. We are a team. As such, we both put effort into the process of understanding and accepting my differences. At times, he helps me work up the courage to advocate for what I need. At other times I educate him on his blind spots in regard to the experience of being disabled.

When I finally began speech therapy, my experiences with CP helped me. I learned early that doing things differently than what was considered 'normal' was okay. I could still do those things and love them. It just took me many years until I was able to apply that philosophy to my speech. Now, as I face fear and hard choices related to CP, I find myself looking back on the journey I have taken through my experiences with my stutter. That journey is one of the things that inspires me to keep trying to talk openly about CP despite the fact that doing so can be difficult.

I have made so much progress in how I think about my CP and my stutter, and I am proud of how far I have come. I know there is never going to be a moment when I reach some kind of perfect enlightenment. There will always be challenges that emerge – some of them physical, others emotional, and many of them societal. I don't think there is one correct way to respond to those challenges; rather, I believe it is an ongoing process of finding my own path, which is what I continue to do.

Stutter naked

Christopher Constantino

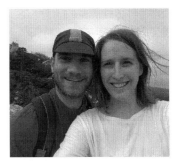

Traveling with my wife.

Stuttering as hardship

At a recent self-help group meeting we had an engaging, and at times provocative, discussion about the *benefit* or *gift* of stuttering. The discussion went the way it usually does, people positioned stuttering as something to grow from. I call this narrative: *stuttering as hardship*. Using the logic of this narrative, stuttering can be a gift in that overcoming it makes us better people, in a what-doesn't-kill-us-makes-us-stronger kind of way. For example, we may learn to be less vain and care less about what others think of us. We may gain empathy and insight into the hidden burdens that all people carry. We might forge close relationships with other people who stutter because we have gone through the same trials and tribulations and, therefore, have a shared history.

Fine. But I wondered if there were other narratives that might add meaning to our stuttered experiences. Is our stuttering only a hardship to be overcome? This suggests that stuttered experiences are, by the logic of the narrative, worse – more difficult, harder, more burdensome – than fluent experiences. It is the very challenge of the stuttered experience that conveys the benefit of growth on a person. If this is all stuttering is, it is not much different than any other challenge. If we did not stutter, we could certainly learn these same lessons elsewhere. Is there not more to our stuttering than this? Is there anything gained from stuttering itself?

Understanding my stuttering

My journey with stuttering has not been one of linear progress over time. I struggled terribly to speak from childhood through adulthood and still do struggle at times. I received some therapy in early grade school but soon dropped out because I did not think it was helping nor did I like being pulled out of class. My primary coping mechanism was to avoid stuttering as much as possible and to grin and bear it when I could not. As I aged, my speech become more effortful and my avoidance behaviours more convoluted.

I have put much distance between where I am now and where I was. This separation allows me to see my stuttering differently. Since I am not thinking about how to be fluent while speaking, my attention is freed up to do other things. I am able to observe my stuttering's effects on others. I am able to offer my stuttering to them, to share it with them. I am now more able to openly and comfortably stutter. I can delight in the surprise of an unexpected stutter or find humour in a particularly goofy manifestation of one. These experiences have led me to see my stutter as a valuable part of myself, something that adds rather than detracts from my speech. I still have moments of struggle and avoidance; the difference is that now I also have moments of joy and delight.

When I stutter, it is not necessarily worse than when I am fluent. It is different. How can I describe this difference? What narratives are available to me? For the most part, there is only one narrative of stuttering widely available to us: the medical model of disability. As discussed by Joshua St. Pierre in Chapter 2, the medical model is a view of disability that categorizes bodies based on norms of functioning, differentiating between those that are 'able-bodied' and those that are 'disabled'. The medical model suggests that norms are statistical matters of fact; everyone who falls outside of a certain number of standard deviations on a bell curve is disabled. However, this is not how disability is actually understood in the real world. For example, by some estimates almost 75% of the US population use some sort of vision correction, yet unaided vision is considered normal. Only one to two percent of the human population has red hair, yet this is not considered disabling. More than 50% of Americans take at least one prescription drug, yet it is viewed as normal to be unmedicated.

The medical model is not completely useless. It is helpful for understanding how our bodies function and for describing disease; however, the medical model often struggles to explain why some differences are considered disabling while others are not. This is where the social model of disability is valuable. The social model suggests that what is and is not disabling has as much to do with societal structures, expectations, and preferences as with standard deviations and bell curves. Someone *becomes* disabled when they cannot be accommodated by society. Disability is not absolute; it is relative to social circumstances. Some people who were not considered disabled in the past may be considered disabled today. For example, before the printing press and in largely agrarian societies, difficulty reading was not a problem, as there was very little to read. However, in modern post-industrial society it can be a large barrier to learning and employment when not accommodated. Conversely, some people who are not considered disabled today may have been considered disabled in the past. For example, there are many modern Americans walking around who, without a doubt, would make very poor traditional hunters (due to physical strength, coordination, body weight, etc.). While these people are considered able-bodied today, they may have found themselves disabled in the past.

If a stutter is spoken in a forest and no one is around...

We never stutter in a vacuum. Bodies necessarily interact with their surroundings. There are well-documented anatomical and physiological differences between those who do and do not have many impairments, stuttering included. However, these differences in themselves do not produce disability. It is only when these differences limit the capability of the individual to function and participate in her society that she becomes disabled. Whether these bodily differences limit participation in society have to with the structure of the society the body inhabits.

We have arrived at the crux of the issue. Does society contribute to our struggles with stuttering? In order to answer this question, some nuance is required. We must define what we mean by stuttering. Stuttering is a neuro-developmental difference that leads to a breakdown in the forward execution of speech sounds produced in the context of language. Stuttering is the underlying feeling, the unhinging of our speech mechanism, the blip, or glitch, that we experience. There are many ways we can react to this misfire; we can silently block, prolong a sound, repeat sounds, syllables, words, or sentences, we can change words, we can stop talking, we can jump up and down, we can smile, we can laugh, we can cry, we can do a flip, or we could bake a potato. But these are not the stutter, these are how we react to and struggle with the stutter. Defined in this way, stuttering cannot be heard by a listener, it is not a sound. It can only be felt by the speaker. What follows the underlying feeling of stuttering is the domain of struggle. Struggle is what the listener hears. Struggle is also a learned behaviour. It typically develops because of avoidance, from an effort not to stutter. It is maintained by habit and often rewarded by society.

No matter how society is structured, my stutter will not go away. The neuroanatomy and neurophysiology that affect my speech mechanism will exist no matter how accommodating my environment. This is not my fault. This insight is actually a benefit of the medical model. Previous models of stuttering would have suggested that we were cursed (religious model), cowardly (moral model), or sexually frustrated (Freudian model). While I might possess a body that produces stuttering, my reaction to my stutter depends on my environment. Society may not control whether or not I am a person who stutters, but it certainly influences whether or not I am a person who struggles when I stutter.

When I think about my stuttering and what it is that I struggle with, it is clear to me that my problem is not that I am unable to, or do not know how to, speak properly. Rather, it is that I do not know how to stutter properly. There is no problem with my articulation or my language skills. I know how to make all my sounds and I have sufficient coordination between my tongue, lips, and vocal folds to move from one sound to another. Yet, because I possess the neuroanatomy and neurophysiology that produces stuttering, my speech is dysfluent. However, dysfluent speech is not necessarily struggled stuttering. The problem is that when I stutter, when I experience the underlying feeling we have labelled as stuttering, I try to stop the stutter. Why do I try not to stutter?

Trying not to stutter

We know from observing the development of stuttering in children that young stutterers can often have very complex and tense stuttering behaviours. This could suggest that, at its onset, there is something fundamentally unsettling about the underlying feeling of stuttering. As young children, we react to this surprising loss of control and unwanted feeling by wrestling with it and attempting to regain control of our speech by force. However, longitudinal studies of children, such as Ehud Yairi and Nicoline Grinager Ambrose's *Early Childhood Stuttering*, have shown that, very often, after this initial period of struggle there is adaptation and stuttering, sometimes quickly, becomes less struggled.

Interestingly, by the time many children who stutter have reached adolescence, their speech behaviours often become struggled again. My own stuttering seems to have followed this pattern. I have few memories of stuttering in grammar and elementary school. I know I did, because I remember speech therapy. But I do not remember thinking much about stuttering. Middle school was different. I remember making decisions not to speak so as to not stutter. I remember deciding there were certain people I could not speak to, pretty girls or popular guys, because I would stutter talking to them. I also remember being mocked, bullied, and punished for stuttering.

This stuttering penalty does not end when we grow up. If anything, it increases as adult experiences are much more consequential than childhood experiences. There is more on the line in a job interview than when navigating the middle school cafeteria. Adults who stutter are discriminated against in their social and professional lives. Through my clinical work and research, I have spoken to people who stutter who have been fired, demoted, physically assaulted, walked out on during dates, told not to speak, laughed at, and insulted for stuttering. We try not to stutter for very good reasons and it has nothing to do with our biology. It is because we are not masochists; we do not enjoy pain. We simply want to live normal lives. When we stutter, normality is denied us.

Both fluent speakers and people who stutter will sometimes suggest that the stutterer's unwillingness to stutter derives from personal weakness rather than societal stigma and discrimination. They suggest that the cure is to have a positive attitude. They position struggle as a psychological issue instead of a sociological one. I, with my co-authors Walter Manning and Susan Nordstrom, refute this idea at length in our 2017 paper on covert stuttering. Many people who stutter are successful navigators of their social worlds. Their avoidances and tricks might not be the healthiest coping mechanisms but, due to society's prejudices, they are often beneficial in the short term. Discrimination against people who stutter is well documented; it is not in our heads. The anxiety that people who stutter have about stuttering has been shown to be a *normal* reaction to stuttering in an unsympathetic society (see Walter Manning and J. Gayle Beck's 2013 articles). In fact, when fluent speech-language pathology graduate students are asked to voluntarily stutter they report similar, if not greater, levels of anxiety. Far from being cowards, people who stutter live daring and courageous lives. Every day they face a world that ridicules them and mocks them. To stutter on a date, in an interview, or on the phone is heroic. People who stutter know what it is to be brave.

The social model of disability does more than shift the locus of disability from the individual's body to the relationship between body and society. It also opens up new questions. If society were more accepting of our speech, what would our stuttering be like? What is it to stutter without stigma? The social model frees stuttering from being defined as the negative opposite of fluency. We can ask a question that is almost unthinkable within the confines of the medical model: what is good about stuttering?

Instead of looking at stuttering as a hardship to overcome and grow from, can we look at it as something to enjoy and delight in? I posed this question to the adult stuttering group. Some members looked at me as if I had a third eye, but some reflected on the question, finding it thought-provoking. We did struggle, however, to come up with satisfying answers. There is not a ready-made narrative for stuttering as anything other than bad, a pathology of the speech mechanism. In our efforts to be positive, the best we have been able to come up with is the *stuttering as hardship* narrative. I'd like to try again at constructing an alternative narrative. I call the narrative: *stuttering as delight*. This has helped me make meaning of my stuttering in valuable ways. You may have had different experiences than I have. I do not expect my ways of making meaning to resonate with everyone, but I hope they provide fodder for your own alternative narratives.

Stuttering as delight

Can stuttering be enjoyed? Stuttering is something for which we are stigmatized and discriminated against. It makes us different from our peers, invites ridicule, and deprives us of our voices. Stuttering is also unpredictable and surprising. We do not stutter on every word nor in every conversation. There is something mysterious and whimsical about stuttering. Stuttering is filled with paradox. We do not often stutter when alone, when we sing, or when we talk to animals. We may not stutter when deeply upset or first thing in the morning. Stuttering is fascinating.

I am reminded of the poem, 'Pied Beauty' by the Jesuit poet Gerard Manley Hopkins, written in 1877:

> Glory be to God for dappled things –
>   For skies of couple-colour as a brindled cow;
>   For rose-moles all in stipple upon trout that swim;
> Fresh-firecoal chestnut-falls; finches' wings;
>   Landscape plotted and pieced – fold, fallow, and plough;
>   And áll trádes, their gear and tackle and trim.
>
> All things counter, original, spare, strange;
>   Whatever is fickle, freckled (who knows how?)
>   With swift, slow; sweet, sour; adazzle, dim;
> He fathers-forth whose beauty is past change:
>   Praise him.

Stuttering is very much a dappled thing, something 'counter, original, spare, strange'. It gives the imagination something to grasp onto, much like a single cloud that breaks up the blue of an otherwise clear sky. A child, armed with her imagination, can turn the cloud into a myriad of wonderful things, but only if its imperfection first exists. As Emma Alpern discussed in Chapter 3, stuttering breaks up the monotony of the conversational soundscape. Stuttering throws a wrench into dialogue. It can turn an ordinary, casual, even banal exchange into something unexpected. For the stutterer, a simple "Good morning" may take as much effort as singing an opera. This prevents us from taking even the simplest dialogue for granted.

The surprise of stuttering, for both listener and speaker, allows it to be the antidote to mundane, trite conversations. How often do we pass our co-workers in the hallway and exchange some pleasantries without even slowing down our pace of walking? We say, "Hi, how're you doing," as we approach. They respond with, "Well, you?" And as we pass them, we finish the exchange with, "Doing great." Successful conversation or wasted breath? There is no exchange of information, no intimacy, the entire interaction has been automatized to the point of absurdity.

Throw some stuttering in and another situation unfolds. My stuttering might cause my fast walking co-worker to slow her pace or maybe even stop walking to engage with me. The forgettable exchange is now replaced by something unique. The co-worker is forced to connect with me. Perhaps we even have meaningful dialogue! Stuttering's ability to change boring situations into novel ones holds true in most conversational interactions. Whether giving a presentation, making a phone call, telling a barista your name, asking a girl out on a date, or asking a bartender for your favourite bourbon, chances are the other person is not expecting stuttering. This instantly changes the nature of the exchange. It becomes new, curious, and singular.

This is not to say that stuttering is better than fluency. People who stutter have been damaged enough by society's preference for fluency over stuttered speech; we do not need to construct the opposite narrative. Rather, stuttering is something different from fluency, something 'fickle' and 'freckled'. In stuttering's difference is beauty. Stuttering adds 'rose-moles' to conversations. The resulting juxtaposition increase their richness.

Delight in intimacy

How do we begin to see the 'pied beauty' of our own stuttering, how do we construct a narrative of *stuttering as delight*? We could start by asking if we have experiences, because we stutter, that we would not have if we did not stutter? The answer is an obvious yes. We can easily name negative experiences: the embarrassment and frustration of not being able to express ourselves, feeling as though we chronically underachieve because of our difficulty communicating, or social and romantic isolation. Can we think of any positive experiences we have gained because we stutter? I am not so much interested in lessons we have learned from *overcoming* our stutters, but in what we have *gained* from stuttering and continuing to stutter.

The most important experience that my stuttering has fostered is *intimacy*. What is required for human intimacy? Whether emotional, sexual, or intellectual, intimacy requires honesty, vulnerability, and sincerity; in a word: nakedness. To be emotionally intimate, you must be willing to share your naked thoughts, feelings, and emotions with another. To be sexually intimate you must be willing to share your naked body, uncovered, and defenseless with another. To be intellectually intimate, you must be willing to share your naked ideas, hypotheses, and insights with another. Intimacy is an act of mutual vulnerability. We make ourselves vulnerable, trusting that the other will do the same. In this mutually vulnerable state we are able to join with the other without false fronts, pretence, or artifice. It is in this state of reciprocated naked, vulnerability, that we truly come to know each other.

The hallmark of stuttering is the temporary inability to move forward through speech, usually described as a *loss of control*. When we stutter, we temporarily lose control, we are temporarily naked. This might sound horrible, like the start of a profoundly bad dream. Hear me out. Repeatedly throughout our day, we are left temporarily defenseless, we are periodically stripped naked. However, the more time we spend naked with others, the more likely we are to experience intimacy. Yes, sometimes this results in embarrassment, mocking, maybe even sunburn! But sometimes people like what they see. We want control over others' perceptions of us. We groom ourselves to look a certain way, try to say the right things at the right times, and self-analyze rather than attend to the moment. Stuttering is a counter to all this distraction. Not only does stuttering disarm us by temporarily wresting away control of our speech but it also serves as a reminder. A reminder to lower our shields, to pay attention to now, and to share ourselves with the person with whom we are speaking.

By stuttering, we can turn vapid social interactions into potentially deep, intimate, and consequential ones. Lowering our guard can cause others to lower theirs. It's a signal to others that the conversational space is safe, we will not be keeping score of decorum or grading them on etiquette. If we allow stuttering to happen, we can invite others to strip and join us. Without all the distraction of fronts and facades we increase our chances of connecting with others and of having worthwhile, meaningful conversations.

The medical model would have us believe that we struggle when we stutter because we have a problem with our bodies. They don't work right. They are pathological. I'd like to offer an alternative explanation: we struggle when we stutter because we have a fear of intimacy. We do not fear intimacy because we are cowards or are deficient. We fear intimacy because we have grown up in a society that stigmatizes the nakedness of our speech. We have been taught by experience that no one wants to see us naked, that we should cover up and hide. We are taught to be embarrassed. The social model of disability allows us to understand our fear of intimacy not as pathology but as a reasonable reaction to a hostile society.

Narrative multitudes

Of course, stuttering is not always a delight. The field of speech-language pathology in the United States was started by people who stutter who did not want to stutter any more. They were tired of struggling to speak and fed up with the ineffective solutions offered by medicine and psychology. The field would not exist if stuttering was always enjoyable. People who stutter would not seek out therapy or spend thousands of dollars on intensive programmes and delayed auditory feedback devices if stuttering was always a lot of fun. The *stuttering as hardship* narrative would not exist if stuttering was easy. No doubt, when I struggle and wrestle with my speech, when all I want to do is express myself, stuttering is far from delightful. Research is clear that, compared to fluent speakers, people who stutter experience a marked reduction in quality of life, personal agency, ability to communicate with others, decreased income, limited job opportunities, and discrimination in their everyday life. None of this is delightful.

Here, I am again reminded of a poem, this time 'Song of Myself', from Walt Whitman's *Leaves of Grass*. Section 51 contains these lines:

> Do I contradict myself?
> Very well then I contradict myself,
> (I am large, I contain multitudes.)

Stuttering, like Whitman, contains multitudes and contradictions. Sometimes it is an ugly thing: robbing us of our voices, our agency, and our freedom. Other times it is a dappled thing, peculiar, surprising, and celebratory. This contradiction need not be resolved.

My stutter can foster intimacy, humility, and show vulnerability. But it does not always accomplish these things. I can also stutter with avoidance, struggle, and anxiety. Rather than foster intimacy, my struggle can become a wedge separating me from the person with whom I am communicating. My avoidance can lessen intimacy and replace it with superficiality. An opportunity for meaningful connection may be replaced with silence. All this contradiction does not prove that stuttering is bad, just that it is a complex and nuanced human behaviour. In other words, stuttering is 'normal'.

Stuttering is not a special human characteristic. The triumph of this contradiction is that it moves stuttering from something special (a pathology that is always bad) to a normal human trait that is more complicated than being simply good or simply bad. There are very few human traits that are unequivocally good. Rather, our unique bodies and minds often give us advantages in some situations and disadvantages in others. Stuttering must be permitted nuance.

Stuttering is no different from other traits. There are times it will be a delight and times it will be a hardship. The problem is that for most of our history, people who stutter have had no choice but to view stuttering as hardship. We can change this. It is not a matter of shifting our attitudes from negative to positive. We cannot simply will ourselves to better lives. However, our experiences of stuttering contain many unacknowledged subtleties and nuances. Joshua Walker, in Chapter 14, calls these unique outcomes. These details of our experience will remain elusive until we have a way of making meaning of them. That is, until we have a narrative that can make use of them.

As long as we are trapped in the stuttering as pathology narrative it is difficult for us to uncover the positive experiences we have had while stuttering. Stuttering as hardship goes some way to exposing some positive experiences. However, these are at most positive effects of *overcoming* stuttering, not positive effects of actually stuttering while speaking. Viewing my stuttering as a delightful source of intimacy has been very helpful in adding meaning to my own experiences.

Perhaps you struggle to make sense of your experiences using my narrative. That is okay. Stutterers are not a homogenous group. We cross every human category imaginable. We are all genders, sexes, races, ethnicities, religions, ages, classes, and sexual orientations. How I add meaning and nuance to my experiences need not be the same way you do. In fact, increasingly diverse narratives help all people who stutter.

The more alternative narratives we have for stuttering the better we will be able to story are experiences in ways that are meaningful and beneficial for us. The social model of disability helps to think outside the box of stuttering as pathology, but it cannot provide alternative narratives. It cannot do the challenging work for us. This is our responsibility as people who stutter. While our narratives will be different, there will be one thing they have in common. They will require us to be naked, to embrace our vulnerability. We cannot re-story our stuttered experiences without allowing our stuttering to exist as it is, exposed, helpless, and nude.

I return to Whitman's 'Song of Myself'. The first line reads:

I celebrate myself, and sing myself

It is my sincere hope that we can learn to celebrate and sing our naked, stuttering selves.

Further reading

Constantino, C.D., Manning, W.H., & Nordstrom, S.N. (2017). Rethinking covert stuttering. *Fluency Disorders, 53*, 26-40.

Hopkins, G.M. (2002). Pied beauty. In *The Major Works* (pp.132-133). New York, NY: Oxford University Press.

Manning, W.H. & Beck, G.J. (2013). The role of psychological processes in estimates of stuttering severity. *Fluency Disorders, 38*(4), 356-367.

Manning, W.H. & Beck, J.G. (2013). Personality dysfunction in adults who stutter: Another look. *Fluency Disorders, 38*(2), 184-192.

Whitman, W. (1855/1993). Song of myself. In *Leaves of Grass* (pp.25-76). New York: Barnes and Nobles Classics.

Yairi, E. & Ambrose, N. (2005). *Early Childhood Stuttering for Clinicians by Clinicians*. Austin, TX: Pro-Ed.

Index